Smoky Mountain Remedies

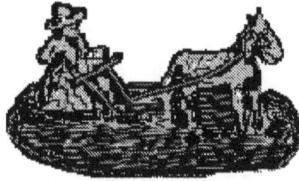

By

Bonnie Trentham Myers

With Glenn Myers and Lyn Myers Boyer

Smoky Mountain Remedies

Copyright © 2007
ISBN 978-0-9727839-6-5
Myers & Myers Publishing
2112 Sentell Circle
Maryville, TN 37803

Myersbon@aol.com

GlennMyers@BellSouth.net

LMBoyer@aol.com

TABLE OF CONTENTS

INTRODUCTION 1
BIRTH AND CHILDCARE 13
BONES, MUSCLES & JOINTS 23
COSMETIC CONCERNS 29
DIGESTIVE ORGANS 41
GENERAL AILMENTS & AFFLICTIONS 53
HEART, BLOOD & BLEEDING 59
INFECTIOUS DISEASES & SANITATION 63
INJURIES & FIRST AID 69
MENTAL CONCERNS, HEADACHES & SLEEP ISSUES 75
PESTS: INSECTS, SNAKES, AND OTHER VERMIN 85
REPRODUCTIVE HEALTH 95
RESPIRATORY AILMENTS 101
SKIN PROBLEMS 113
VETERINARY CONCERNS 127
VISION AND HEARING 131
GENERAL REMEDIES 135

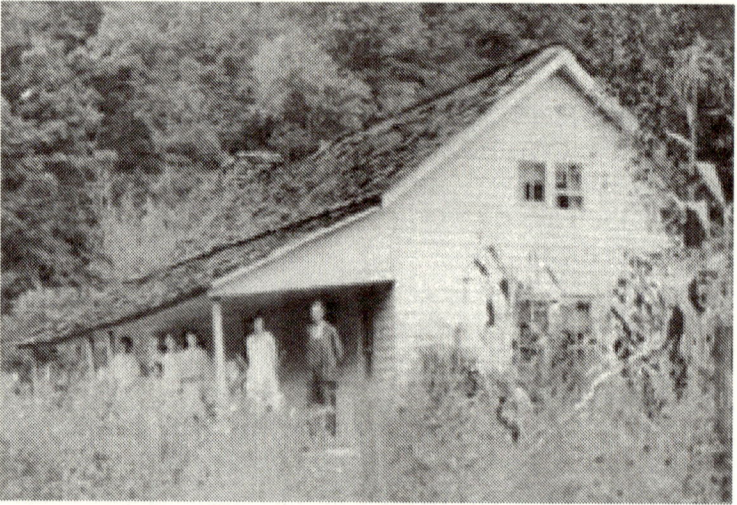

My home place in what is now the Great Smoky Mountains National Park. (L-R) Mary Jane Ogle Carr Trentham, Bonnie Trentham Myers, Gladys Trentham Russell Yeaton, Kate Trentham Stogner, Sam E. Trentham, Verna Trentham, Noah H. Trentham.

INTRODUCTION

When I was a child growing up on a farm that was to become part of the Great Smoky Mountains National Park, I recall seeing a doctor for treatment only two or three times. One time, I fell from our porch while swinging on the chain of our porch swing. The gashes I received in my leg were quite deep. My dad took me to Sevierville, where Dr. McMahan put some kind of metal pieces (probably metal staples) in my legs to put me back together.

Although I remember seeing doctors very few times, there were many times members of my family could have benefited from medical care. However, seeing a doctor in those days was generally out of the question. There were few doctors, and money was scarce.

When illness or injury struck our family, we used whatever we had. Unlikely as it seems today, when my sister Gladys (Trentham Russell Yeaton) cut the bone in her little finger so that it appeared to be hanging by one small piece of skin, she did not see a doctor. My Dad merely went to the smokehouse to get a bucket of varnish. He applied a small amount to each side of the severed bone, and he stuck it back together. Then, he wrapped a rag around it, and waited for it to grow back. My sister, now 90, recently wiggled that finger for me. It looked as if nothing had ever happened to it. I wonder how using varnish would do today to glue broken bones back together.

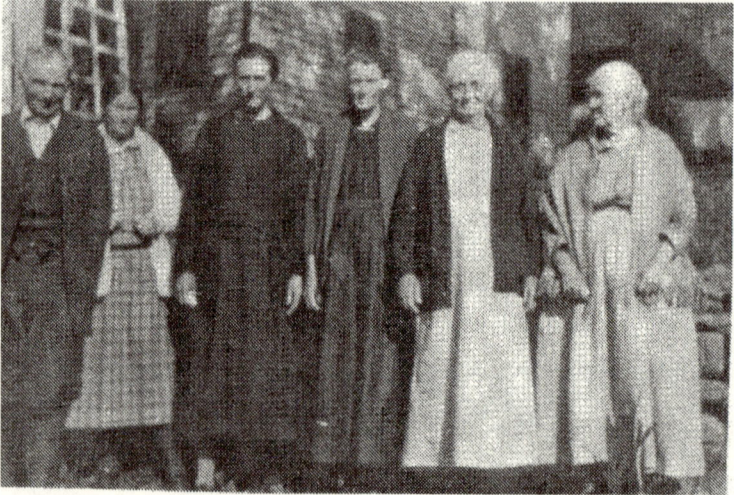

Dr. Hoffman taught classes in midwifery. Shown are, from left to right: Dr. Hoffman, Laura Whaley, Mary Jane Ogle Carr Trentham (my mother), Polly Whaley, Celia Ownby, and Sarah Cole.
(Courtesy of *Velma Lamons*)

My other sister, Kate (Trentham Stogner), really needed to see a doctor when both of her feet were badly crushed beneath trolley car wheels when she was a child. I do not remember what treatment my parents provided, but today at age 92, doctors say they do not understand how she has been able to walk on those badly injured feet all these years.

Until we moved out of what was to become the Park in 1933, we were never even close to real medical doctors. I can only recall one, Dr. Hoffman, who made trips into area homes and also taught a group of women, including my mother, Mary Jane Ogle Carr Trentham, how to perform services as midwives in our community.

In 1922, Pi Beta Phi School opened the Jennie Nicol Memorial Hospital in a house in Gatlinburg. It was really little more than a small clinic for the students there. I do not remember that anyone could have stayed there for more intensive care than they could receive at home. The nurse, Miss Marjorie Chalmers, also served the community to some extent. She spent many years at this clinic, and later wrote a book called *Better I Stay,* describing her experiences.

Dr. John Ogle was generally recognized as a good physician in the Sevierville and Pigeon Forge area. We children enjoyed repeating a remark he was famous for saying. "Take a dose (pronounced dauce) of salts followed by oil, and if you are not better in the morning, call me." That meant Epsom salts and castor oil. We enjoyed mispronouncing the word "dose" and, of course, we hated both the Epsom salts and castor oil treatment he prescribed for nearly every ailment.

Certain people in the community were known as healers. In addition to knowing herbal remedies, they knew verses or chants that were supposed to cure illnesses. Some healers silently quoted the following verse while touching the patient: "My loaf in my lap; my penny in my purse. Thou are now the better; I am none the worse." (They accepted only a penny for their services.) They believed healers were required to walk barefoot on the earth or on

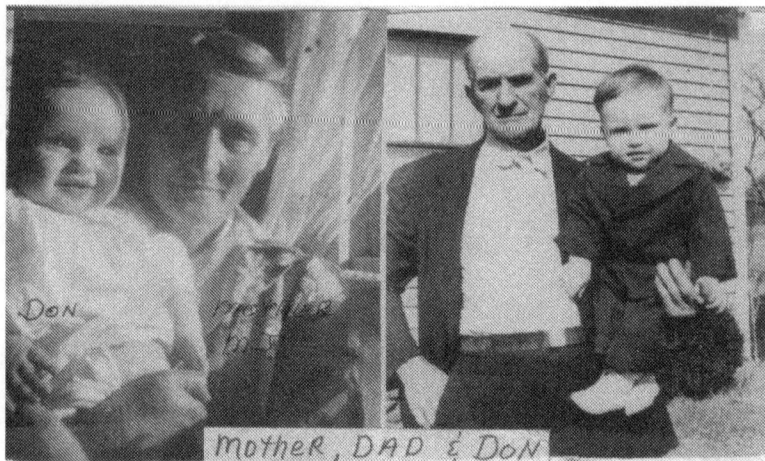

My parents, Mary Jane Ogle Carr Trentham and Noah H. Trentham each holding Donald Trent Myers, my first child. They were considered healers in our community.

the dewy grass in the sunlight to renew their energy.

When the circus came to town in Pigeon Forge, snake oil merchants hawked their wares. Unbelievably, some of it may really have helped. They often mixed red pepper in mineral oil. Some research today indicates the capsaicin in red pepper may have reduced pain. Sometimes they used alcohol, which would make an individual feel better for a while. Camphor and turpentine were other ingredients used in these mixtures.

Primitive conditions made it difficult for anyone with a serious medical problem. Early surgery was done amid screams and tremendous pain. Whiskey was often the best way to prepare for medical procedures. Ether was available for anesthesia in my early days. When not properly monitored, ether could prove disastrous.

My parents were the medical experts for our community. As mentioned previously, my mother was trained as a midwife. After her death, we found records showing that she helped to deliver 195 babies without losing a mother or a baby. At a fee of only $5, many times after helping to deliver a baby, she returned to the family's home with clothing or other items they needed.

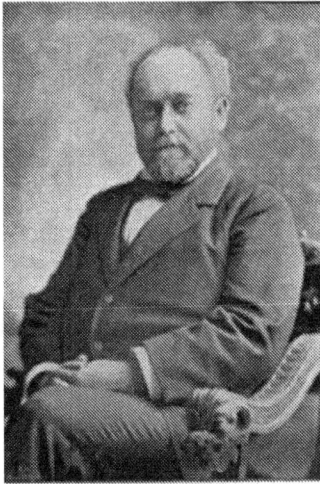

My dad, Noah Trentham, learned about treatments for various ailments, and our neighbors asked him when they had medical concerns. When a question arose that my parents could not answer, they referred to an old copy of "Dr. Pierce," as they called it. I have since learned that it was probably *The People's Common Sense Medical Advisor in Plain English*, written in 1895 by Dr. Ray Vaughan Pierce. Despite my parents' limited formal education, they were able to determine what Dr. Pierce prescribed for various illnesses and conditions.

I recently ran across a copy of this book. A review of the contents shows a clear attempt to sell his rather long list of proprietary medicines, called *materia medica*, and to make readers aware of his large Invalids' Hotel and Surgical Institute in Buffalo, New York. The book also contained many testimonials from all over the country describing the incredible results of treatment derived from the medicines and the Institute. One of those testimonials is shown below. I particularly enjoyed reading why the husband seemed pleased with his wife's progress.

BRONCHITIS AND LUNG DISEASE.

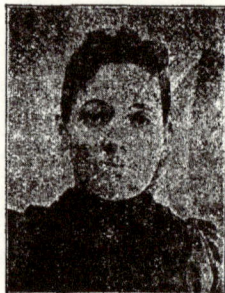

Mrs. Neal, of Crockett Mills, Tenn., had an attack of measles, followed by bronchitis and pneumonia. Her husband writes, "I feel gratified with the effect of your wonderful medicine. I can recommend it to anybody, and feel I am doing them justice. My wife was not able to perform her household duties for six months. She has used two bottles of 'Golden Medical Discovery,' and is now able to do all her work. I think it the finest medicine in the world, and I am, gratefully,

Your life-long friend,
J.B. NEAL.

We did not mean use each remedy. However, we were aware of many of them. To my knowledge, no one in my family was ever

6

bitten by a snake. We did not use chants, charm warts, or carry buckeyes to guard against arthritis.

Not all remedies worked, but they were usually easy to use and, of course, inexpensive. Our remedies are scientifically unproven, and they should not today take the place of professional medical evaluation and treatment. Some remedies can be dangerous for people taking certain prescription medications. And, some are now considered just plain dangerous.

Possibly, because of my family history, I inherited a life-long interest in healing and alternative medical treatments. Over the years, I have collected many remedies, both from the Smoky Mountains and outside. No matter what the ailment, I have always had a remedy to suggest. In addition, I worked at the Gatlinburg Medical Center with the late Dr. Ralph Shilling and Dr. Terrell Tanner, and later I retired from Blount Memorial Hospital in Maryville, Tennessee. I must say that occasionally my home remedies and ideas about alternative treatments were the source of some friction with the doctors with whom I worked.

Several months ago, my granddaughter, Amanda Myers, asked me to write down for her all my home remedies. She did not specify that they be old, new, or in-between. I had already included many of them in my first book, *Best Yet Life and Lore of the Smokies*. However, with her request and the suggestion from others that I share my remedies, I am compiling, with the help of my son and daughter, the remedies I have collected over the past 85 years.

This is not a comprehensive listing of home remedies or herbal supplements; there are many sources of information on those topics. I have attempted to limit my discussion to those that were used or have been used by friends and family in and around the Smoky Mountains. However, because I have taken bits and pieces from many different sources over the years, I have inserted a few that came from other locations.

As we began this project, I asked friends and neighbors about remedies they remembered as children. I was both delighted and surprised by the variety of treatments they related. I would like to thank each of them for their contributions. This project has been very enlightening and enjoyable for me, and I hope it brought back some pleasant memories for those who provided me some of their old family remedies.

I also hope readers will find these remedies and the stories that go with them interesting and perhaps entertaining. It is not my intent to present these for your use. If you should try something I have included, please be aware that you do so at your own risk. Over the years, I have used many of them with no adverse effects. I cannot vouch for all of them.

As we begin, I will list some of the very colorful descriptions and (mis)pronunciations for medical terms and physical impairments that many of us used. I have often said that if it was possible to mispronounce something, we did it. In some cases, I have included pronunciation guides.

- Backset – relapse of an illness
- Bad disease – syphilis (with vocal emphasis on the word *bad*)
- Beal – an infection: "My skin has bealed."
- Belly band – a cloth fastened around a newborn to prevent an umbilical rupture
- Bitters – herbs (pronounced *yarbs*)
- Blood stopper – one who uses the *Bible* verse Ezekiel 16:6 to stop blood
- Bloody flux – dysentery
- Bold hives – potentially fatal illness in infants caused by hives
- Breath killer – something used to stop bad breath
- Burn doctor – one who blows fire out of a burn or who performs the burn ceremony
- Corruption – pus: "There is corruption in the sore on my foot."
- Courage – sex drive: "Her husband lost his courage."
- Creel – a sprain
- Fall off – weight loss: "I fell off a sight bad."
- Far'·ed – forehead (I did not realize until I saw the word in print that we had been mispronouncing it.)

- Fleshy – slightly overweight
- Flux – diarrhea
- Gald – heat rash: "I'm so galded [gal-ded] I can scarcely walk."
- Gravel – gallstones
- Hippoed – sickly feeling or pretending to be sick
- The itch – scabies or seven-year-itch
- Jake leg – a clumsy or palsied walk
- Kernels – swollen glands
- Mare's carry – When a baby was overdue, they superstitiously said the mother had passed under a mare's neck. A long pregnancy coincided with the gestation period of a mare.
- Nature – sex drive: "My nature [is] all tore up."
- Nuss - a corruption of the word nurse. When your mother, grandmother, or a favorite aunt asked you to come sit on her lap, she said, "Come, let me *nuss* you." I have not heard the word used in more than 75 years.
- Out of heart – depressed
- Peaked – (pronounced as two words, peak–kid) Appearing sick: "She looked mighty peaked to me."
- Pert – (pronounced peert) lively, feeling good
- Phthisic – Having asthma or possibly tuberculosis. This word was used in spelling bees at our schools.
- Pieded – (pronounced as two words, pie·ded) spotted skin
- Piles - hemorrhoids
- Pone - a raised swelling
- Poorly - not well: "I am feelin' a mite poorly."

- Pumpknot - a bump or raised swelling, usually on the head: "He got a pumpknot on his head when he fell."
- Puny - appearing or feeling ill: "She looks a mite puny."
- Quare - (rhymes with square - probably a mispronunciation of *queer*.) a term used to describe a person who is unusual. i.e. "He's a mite quare."
- Risin' - carbuncle or boil: "I have a risin' on my arm."
- Scald head - scabs or sores on one's head
- Scours - diarrhea: "He had the scours."
- Sinking spell - fainting spell: "She had a sinkin' spell."
- Smotherin' - breathing difficulty
- Sore eyes - conjunctivitis or pink eye
- Stove – to jam up a joint, often in the fingers or toes: "I stove up my finger when I hit the wall."
- Strutted - swollen: "My ankle strutted."
- Stump water - water caught in the cavity of a stump. I was told stump water would remove my freckles. I never actually tried it.
- Swimmy headed - dizzy: "I felt all swimmy headed."
- Touched (pronounced teched - rhyming with fetched) mentally unsound: "He's a mite teched in the hā·id [head]."
- Weak trembles - quivering or weakness in the legs
- Yarbs - herbs

Other comments sometimes used:
- "I ain't much stout yet, but the spells ain't common."
- "I had such miseries -My nerves all tore up."
- "I felt like I'd been kicked in the head by a mule."
- "I felt sight on earth bad."

11

· "It'll quore (cure) what ails ye."

Categories of conditions or ailments are included in each of the next few chapters. In each category are some related conditions and some of the remedies I have collected for treatment or prevention. The last chapter of the book is a listing of our most commonly used remedies. The index provides a cross-reference for both conditions and remedies.

BIRTH AND CHILDCARE

Superstition played a part in the everyday life of many in the mountains - including beliefs about birth and pregnancy. Some people believed that the bed on which a visiting newborn was first laid would be the next one to produce a new baby. Soon after Mrs. Guilford Tyler (Thelma), one of our church members, had a new baby, she came to visit me. She intentionally placed her baby on our bed, and then said to me, "Now, you will have the next baby." I doubt there was any connection, but my daughter Lyn came along a few months later.

On New Year's Day of 1948, about the same time, I went with my husband to visit his parents in Wear's Valley. My father-in-law was furious with me. He said it was bad luck for a woman to visit on that day. He was not going to let me in his house. [Conversely, it was good luck for a man to visit.]

A few months later, when my husband and I announced that I was pregnant, he reminded me that bad luck was supposed to occur as a result of that visit. I assured him that had nothing to do with it.

In this chapter I have included treatments, beliefs and stories related to children and the care they received.

13

CASTOR OIL – When we were growing up, our mother always gave us castor oil, which was the all-purpose preventative and treatment for most childhood ailments. Most old-timers today recall that no matter what ailment they had, a dose of castor oil was administered. We often did not tell Mother if we were sick, because we did not want her to reach for the handy castor oil bottle. I really do not remember that we used a lot of castor oil in my house, because we simply did not mention an illness if we could avoid it.

The usual dosage was one drop to 99 drops of water. Now, I have learned that the castor plant contains the third most poisonous substance in the world. I bet many children back then would have appreciated knowing that piece of information.

CATS – Many believed that cats suck the breath out of a baby. I once found our cat standing over my daughter when she was a baby. I do not know that the cat was sucking her breath, but it had its mouth on hers. The cat did not have that opportunity again.

CHILDBIRTH – Primitive women used the old-fashioned birthing stool when delivering babies. The stool appears to have enabled them to bear children with less fuss and pain than more modern methods. As a midwife, my mother did not use birthing stools. Around us, only women who did their own deliveries used them. However, I have been interested to see that some women are electing to use midwives and birthing stools today.

For some reason, the first command before a baby's delivery was to "boil some water!" I never knew exactly why. There were no utensils to sterilize. Of course, the midwife could use warm water to wash her hands and to have bath water for the new baby. Maybe it gave nervous fathers something to keep themselves occupied.

If the delivery was prolonged, the mother was sometimes instructed to drink a bottle of castor oil to speed up the delivery. My mother carried a product called Nux Vomica in her medical bag to induce vomiting during a difficult delivery. I learned this product is still available today.

Some used an unusual method to assist in the delivery of a baby. A small amount of powdered snuff [tobacco] was placed on a plate. When it was nearly time for delivery, someone would say, "It's time to sniff her." At that time, someone blew the snuff into the expectant mother's face. Her reaction would be so violent as to bring forth the baby.

A new mother was kept perfectly quiet in bed for at least ten days after the birth of a baby. This practice was supposed to allow the organs to "knit back." In 1942, I was a victim of that treatment with my first baby. On the tenth day, I was so weak that I had to be turned over in bed. With the other two babies, I was up and walking around very quickly.

CHILDCARE – Women had few of the modern conveniences for babies. I have listed below some of the ingenious ways mountain women dealt with some of the childcare issues for which we have more modern solutions.

- All diapers were cloth, usually made from torn bed sheets. Diapers were boiled in a large black pot over a fire after each use.

- A piece of pork rind sometimes served as a teething ring. One end of a string was tied to the pork rind, and the other end was tied to the baby's big toe. If the baby started to choke on the rind, he would kick his feet and legs, which would pull the rind out of his mouth.

- Long before babysitters, mountain women who had to go outside to do chores, found a way to keep their babies out of trouble. When leaving the little one alone in the house, mothers raised the bed leg and set it on the baby's dress tail. This may account for the fact that baby boys usually wore dresses for several months.

- Many women believed that allowing a baby to continue nursing prevented pregnancy. Young children, even up to age six, were known to ask mothers to meet them behind the door for a feeding.

- Baking soda or cornstarch was used to bathe babies.

- Before today's salves for diaper rash came on the market, milk of magnesia was sometimes applied.

· To control bed-wetting, parents used one or more of the following remedies:

- One teaspoon of honey every night before bed.

- A tea made of corn silks.

- No fluids after 5:00 P.M.

- Chewing cinnamon bark.

COD LIVER OIL – Many children were given daily doses of cod liver oil, which was supposed to prevent just about every childhood disease. I talked to a neighbor who said she had to take cod liver oil every day until age 17. She demonstrated how she held her nose while taking it. Another neighbor, who had eight brothers and sisters, said he and all his siblings lined up daily to take cod liver oil mixed with turpentine. It is interesting that recently a top doctor endorsed cod liver oil as a blood thinner, saying that it also protects the heart.

COLDS – Various poultices were used for children with severe colds, sore throats, and chest congestion. For infants with a chest cold or sore throat, parents made a poultice of mustard powder mixed with honey. They added flour and lard or vegetable oil to make a mixture like a biscuit or pancake dough. The mixture was flattened out like a pancake and spread directly on the chest or throat. Then, they covered it with a cloth and left it on overnight. The flour kept it from being too hot for a baby. For older children and adults, the flour, used to reduce the heat of the mustard, may not have been necessary.

For sore throat, some parents melted salty butter and poured it into a child's throat as he or she went to bed. They were usually well the next morning.

COLIC - To cure colic, some parents used a tea made of ground ivy, which I have heard contains a mild tranquilizer. Or, parents gave infants weak teas made from dill, fennel, or catnip. Some used a very small amount of paregoric.

CRADLE CAP – (eczema) To cure cradle cap, mothers were instructed to massage into the scalp a small amount of warmed sweet oil (olive oil) mixed with an infusion of evening primrose.

FEEDING BABIES - Long before blenders and baby foods came along, mothers practiced a custom we find disgusting today. The mother chewed the food and transferred it to the infant's mouth. If the infant was extremely hungry, the mother passed her index finger back and forth across her mouth to show the crying baby she was chewing as fast as possible. That gesture seemed to pacify the child.

If a newborn baby cried for food before the mother began producing milk, the mother often tied a lump of sugar into a clean white cloth and then quickly dipped the cloth into water. This combination, called a "sugar tit," was given to the infant to suck. If available, the milk of very young and tender fresh corn was also used as a substitute for mother's milk.

In very early days, baby food or gruel was made using one teaspoon of slippery elm powder mixed with one pint of boiling water and powdered sugar. This was mixed slowly. When it was flavored with cinnamon or nutmeg, it made a wholesome sustaining food for infants. Some said that it is as nutritious as oatmeal.

HIVES – If a baby developed hives, parents often rubbed catnip on its skin to provide relief.

MASTITIS - Women sometimes had what they called "milk weed" or the "weed" after giving birth. This was mastitis or inflammation of the breasts. Treatments included placing hot compresses on the affected breast or taking doses of propolis, echinacea, or poke.

PREDICTING A BABY'S SEX – People often wanted to know the sex of a baby before it was born. Long before ultrasound (and ultrasound expense), mountain folk used unique methods to determine the sex. They claimed to be able to predict the sex of a baby by looking into the eyes of the mother-to-be. If a red streak was at the 4 o'clock location, they said the baby was a boy. If a streak was at eight o'clock, it was a girl. This process was called iridology.

A pendulum was also used to predict the sex of unborn babies. Slipping a ring on a piece of string about 20 inches long, someone held both ends of the string over the abdomen of an expectant mother. The ring was allowed to swing like a pendulum. It was supposed to work best if the expectant mother was lying down. If the ring swung in a straight line, the baby was said to be a boy. If the ring swung in a circle, the baby was said to be a girl. (Note the symbols used to determine a baby's sex.)

A later method used to determine the sex of a baby was to drop some of the expectant mother's urine from the first specimen in the morning into some Drano. If it turned brown or golden, the baby was said to be a girl. If the Drano turned green, it was supposed to be a boy. I have known of this being correct. Of course, the chances are 50/50 that it will be.

PREGNANCY – There was no prenatal care in my early years, but by the time I was married, we consulted doctors during pregnancy. There was no discussion about diet or exercise. The only thing I remember about treatment was that doctors asked pregnant women to bring them urine samples. I remember taking urine samples to my doctors frequently. It seems like I was doing that every two or three days. I do not have a clue as to what they were doing with it. Maybe research?

SPRING TONIC - Every spring, children all over our area were given a spring tonic to rev up our tired blood after the cold winter months. Spring tonics were said to make your blood rise like the sap in the trees. Recipes varied from family to family, and often they were quite foul tasting. At our house, we were always given sulfur mixed with molasses (called 'lasses.) The dose was one teaspoon of the mixture every day for five days. It did not taste bad. In fact, I liked it.

Other parents insisted on more exotic concoctions. Many used spicewood twigs, sometimes mixed with fresh violet leaves or dried boneset leaves (a wild plant found in the Smokies.) Some used alfalfa as a tonic. If the tonic tasted really awful, compassionate mothers added a little honey. However, the general feeling was that the worse it tasted, the better it was for you.

THROAT OBSTRUCTION - If a child had an obstruction in the throat or windpipe, it was lifted by the feet with its head downward, and someone administered a sharp blow between the shoulder blades.

THRUSH – Perhaps the most unusual treatment I recollect came with the treatment of thrush, a yeast infection in the mouth found

21

most often in infants or toddlers. When an infant or adult contracted this infection, the suggested treatment was to find a person whose father had died before they were born. Having this individual blow into the infected mouth was supposed to cure the infection. Strange as it sounds, I remember people in Wear's Valley talking about this treatment without a hint of skepticism.

BONES, MUSCLES & JOINTS

I remember when I was a child, a woman we called Aunt Donnie lived near us. She was so stooped that, as she walked, her face was parallel to the ground. When she passed our house, she would turn her head and look in my direction. Despite her obviously uncomfortable condition, she would always smile. I still remember her beautiful smile to this day.

We did not know the importance of calcium or the benefits of Vitamin D. Treatments for muscle and skeletal problems were often limited to trying to set broken bones and reducing pain when it occurred. There was little in the way of prevention and cure, and the hard work contributed to muscle pain and injuries. Bone, muscle, and joint problems were common, particularly in older folks. Below, I have listed remedies I have collected that were supposed to help or prevent these conditions.

ARTHRITIS and **RHEUMATISM** - Because we referred to both arthritis and rheumatism as "rhum-atis," I have combined the two. The accent was on the first syllable with a quick "a-tis" following. It was pronounced a little like the word *remedies* (**room·a·tis.**)

I sometimes heard old-timers describe arthritis as being "hate in the bones!" I took that to mean that if people held hatred in their heart, they could expect to get arthritis.

Very early treatments for rheumatism, inflamed joints, included using leeches. If the leeches did not soon adhere to the skin, milk or sweetened water were applied. The leeches remained on the skin until they naturally fell off. After the treatment, the skin was dusted with flour. Joint pain was common enough that many remedies were touted to relieve it. The following were suggested.

- Old-timers believed that carrying a buckeye would prevent arthritis and rheumatism. (Some coal miners would never enter a mine without a buckeye in their pockets.)

- A favorite remedy still used today is to eat gold raisins soaked in gin. Mix and let them soak for four days; then eat eight or ten each day.

- Apply a mixture of a large amount of camphor dissolved in whiskey to sore areas.

- Carry a fresh raw potato in your pocket until it shrivels up. When it shrivels, replace it. This was believed to draw out the acids or poisons that cause muscle and joint pain.

- Eat a raw potato three times a day.

- Drink tea made of chili peppers, burdock, or alfalfa leaves or seeds.

- Mix equal parts of apple cider vinegar and honey, and take one tablespoon every day.

- As we started shopping in grocery stores, we found one very special remedy for muscle and joint discomfort. It was our old standby, Certo, which was used to make jams and jellies. We drank one tablespoon morning and evening in unsweetened grape juice. It unlocked fingers and hands, which had been locked with arthritis.

- Another old remedy is to add enough water to cover two ounces of cinnamon sticks and three ounces of fresh ginger. Bring the water to a boil over medium heat, and boil until the water is reduced to half. Drink a cupful three times a day.

I buy all my honey from Howard Kerr, a beekeeper and a former president of the beekeepers' association. He told me a story about his mother's arthritis that is hard to believe. One time the bees in one of his bee gums became ill so that he took that gum to his mother's house to prevent infecting his other bees.

He set the bees in his mother's yard close to her clothesline. Apparently, the flapping of drying clothes irritated them. When she hung her clothes on the line, she was stung a number of times. This prompted her to call Howard to demand that he move his bees.

Several days passed before Howard could go to her house. When he arrived to pick up the bees, his mother was standing guard in front of them. "Don't you dare move those bees!" she said. Howard could not imagine what prompted such a change of heart. It seems that her extremely bad case of arthritis had improved so much that she decided the bee stings had relieved her pain. She was able to move her fingers and button her clothes after many years of suffering. I do not know if this is a treatment I would want to try. I understand that bee venom is now sold for a variety of purposes, however.

Other less extreme treatments for arthritis are:

- Spend 30 minutes each day pulling on an imaginary rope in all directions. I understand that remedy has taken patients out of wheel chairs.

- Many people have used WD-40 for arthritis, but the company has not endorsed the practice. I suspect they do not discourage purchasing their product for this purpose, however. I understand they published an article that says WD-40 has nothing in it to hurt you.

- Edgar Cayce, the well-known psychic, said no one who would rub joints with peanut oil need ever fear arthritis.

BACK AND MUSCLE PAIN – Before chiropractors and orthopedic doctors, those experiencing backache mixed turpentine and sugar and applied the mixture to sore muscles.

Beginning in the very early 1900's, Doan's Backache Kidney Pills were heavily advertised in newspapers and later on radio and television. Somewhere along the way, because of government questions, the company dropped the reference to kidneys. The most recent information I have is that the government questions the reference to backache as well.

26

- One old-time remedy for back and muscle pain is to apply a plaster made of mustard. The heat probably makes the muscles feel better.

- Many extol the merits of soaking sore muscles in Epsom salts.

- I have a hard time believing this one, but here it is. Just soak sore muscles in buttermilk.

- Some believe magnets really help sprains and general well-being. Just to see, I have slept on them and sometimes wore them in my shoes. I did not note any difference.

GOUT - Apply hot vinegar mixed with salt four times a day. Or, eat any kind of fresh or canned cherries. I have now learned that cherries contain minute amounts of a natural sedative phytochemical - whatever that is.

PIGEON TOES - Today the condition is called in-toeing. This term, and others we used, may sound derogatory today, but they were the only names we knew. For children with this condition, our remedy was to have them sleep with the right shoe on the left foot and the left shoe on the right foot for a few weeks.

LAMENESS - Mix one-tablespoon turpentine, one egg yolk, and one-tablespoon apple cider vinegar. Rub in well. This remedy has been used both for animals and people.

LEG CRAMPS – The oldest remedies are bathing legs in apple cider vinegar, wrapping them in warm towels, or spraying them with very warm water. Some say to put feet in cold water to relieve leg cramps.

Another interesting remedy is to squeeze hard on the upper lip. When I was dancing with members of our senior citizens' group, we occasionally had cramps in our legs. I usually suggested that they stand three feet from a wall with feet flat on the floor and bend the body toward the wall. This usually helped.

More recently, I heard the following unbelievable remedy. After hearing it a number of times, I read it in a health periodical quoting two people who seemed to have all their marbles. Put a bar of soap, preferably non-perfumed, under your lower legs while sleeping. They say to put the soap under the sheet, but I put mine in a sock. I am still dubious, but I have tried it with some success. It may be the placebo effect.

SPRAINS - Dip a brown paper bag in apple cider vinegar and wrap around a sprained ankle to relieve the pain and swelling. We have also soaked sprained ankles in very warm water and Epsom salt. Doctors today suggest that you use an ice pack for the first 24 hours and apply heat afterwards.

COSMETIC CONCERNS

Looking our best was just as important then as it is today. There were few products on the market to help with the process, but we were careful with hair and skin. I do not recall women in our area using makeup until about the time I was married. I heard tell of using flour for powders, but it was too white I would think. I cannot recall even using lipstick until after my high school days.

Even until the late 1930's, mountain women wore long hair. It was usually gathered and wrapped around their heads in buns. Braided buns were very common. According to the preachers, a woman's hair was her "glory." In the 1920's my mother-in-law, Ida Headrick Myers, "bobbed" (cut) her hair. There was discussion about "turning her out" of her church in Wears Valley. My two older sisters had to wear long hair. I do not know how I escaped, but my hair was never long.

ACNE - Many people today are paying as much as $150 per month for topical acne treatments when our good ole propolis (from beehives) mixed with brandy costs about $20. Having seen miraculous results within a week, I think we have the greatest acne cure in the world. While I prefer the propolis treatment, those who did not have it applied a paste of baking soda mixed with a small amount of water to the affected area.

29

Another remedy is to apply a mixture of lemon juice and a well-beaten egg white. The remainder can be chilled for later use. Echinacea has also been used both orally and applied to the skin. Today, some use a dab of preparation H.

AGING - We were told that aging starts in our toes. Maybe that is good if it goes to our brains last. We were also told that if we pulled out one gray hair, seven more would take its place.

Mountain women did not like to age any more than women do today. Their methods may not have been as scientific - or as expensive - but they were used with enthusiasm and hope. Many grandmothers never had gray hair because they rinsed their long hair in boiled sage, rosemary, or chamomile. Chamomile was also used to highlight blond hair. Other dyes were made from onionskins, walnut hulls, and hickory bark. My grandmother, Mary Ann Ogle, combed coffee into her hair for color. Others rubbed the inside of the peel of pawpaws (our locally grown bananas) on their hair to return its natural color.

AGE SPOTS (BROWN SPOTS OR LIVER SPOTS) – I have run across a number of remedies suggested for age spots, but staying out of the sun seems to be the only real solution. Topical remedies include applying the following items to age spots each day for a few weeks: castor oil, buttermilk, lemon juice, vitamin E, the inside of an orange peel, or hydrogen peroxide.

Mixtures used to remove age spots include applying one teaspoon of onion juice mixed with two teaspoons of vinegar or applying equal parts of honey and yogurt for 30 minutes daily for a few weeks. I have rubbed vinegar on the purple spots on my legs and was surprised how the color faded.

BALDNESS – My Trentham relatives, including my father and both my sons, inherited a gene for baldness. I do not remember any of them actually attempting to grow more hair, but I have collected some remedies over the years.

- Some mountain men applied previously used cylinder oil for baldness. I was never acquainted with anyone who used it, but I heard about its use.

- Mix one teaspoon rubbing alcohol and one teaspoon Vaseline. Apply the mixture to the scalp twice a week at bedtime and leave on overnight.

- Rub onto the scalp a tea made of peach leaves or a mixture of two tablespoons of moonshine and one-half teaspoon cayenne pepper.

- Break sections of a grape vine and set in a glass. When the juice drains out of the vine, massage the liquid into the scalp each day for 30 days.

- Rub on the scalp a mixture of castor oil and enough alcohol to dilute it.

- Add five drops of iodine to one pint of water and two teaspoons of baking soda. Massage well three times a day for three weeks. During this time, wash the scalp with mild soap.

- Add six drops of iodine and one teaspoon of honey to one pint of apple cider vinegar. Apply every day for fourteen days. Use mild soap.

- Massage with aloe twice a day until you see progress or give up on the idea.

BATHING – As I was growing up, we made our soap in large kettles out in the yard. We used fat from slaughtered hogs and lye, which came from ashes saved from our fireplace. Making soap was an involved process, but the product worked very well.

Each day we washed thoroughly using a washbasin. Every Saturday night we took turns bathing in our large galvanized washtub behind the warm cook stove in our kitchen. We carried very cold water from the springhouse and heated it in the large reservoir of our wood-burning stove. The stove held many gallons of water, which were heated as we cooked.

When we moved out of what is now the Park and began purchasing more items in stores, we bought soap at my cousin Robert Pickle's Grocery Store in Pigeon Forge. I remember that my mother always bought Ivory soap. Each time I smell Ivory today, I think of her.

BREATH FRESHENERS – Even as late as the 1960's, my family used Sen-Sen, a product that I understand is still on the market. It was called a breath perfume as well as a candy or confection. First produced in the 1800's, Sen-Sen was not made in our area, but it was sold in many small stores around the country. Less exotic breath fresheners are parsley, vinegar, birch, wintergreen, chamomile, bayberry or peppermint.

CELLULITE – I remember that a family member had a bad case of cellulite. The old remedy was simply to rub the area daily with some kind of oil. When millions of women today spend millions of dollars on pricy products in hopes of smoothing out those lumps and bumps, the cure may be right in their kitchens.

DANDRUFF – Our early treatment for dandruff was to rub salt on the scalp for a short time and then to shampoo. We sometimes applied apple cider vinegar and left it on the scalp for one hour, or we shampooed three times a week using white vinegar as a rinse. Some used a mixture of one tablespoon of witch hazel and one teaspoon of lemon juice. This was left on the scalp for one hour before rinsing and shampooing.

DENTAL CARE - We never had dentists until the late 1930's, and we were not familiar with preventive care such as flossing and fluoride treatments. In fact, many fully expected to lose their teeth as they grew older.

We brushed our teeth using toothbrushes made from tender birch sticks approximately five inches long. We removed about one inch of bark from one end of the wood and chewed that end of the stick until the fiber broke apart. When the fiber flattened into a circle, we used the circular fiber for our toothbrushes. Goose quills were used for toothpicks.

Because packaged toothpaste was not available to us when I was a child, we brushed with a mixture of baking soda and salt. The taste is very pleasant once you find the right proportions and get used to it. We sometimes used it instead of toothpaste when my children were growing up.

When we developed tooth decay, filling cavities was not an option. The following remedies were suggested for toothache. Place two cloves in the jaw. Chew a bit of the cloves to release the juice. Or, split a raisin in half. Cover it with black pepper, and place it on the tooth.

For gum problems, we rinsed the mouth with a weak solution of salt and vinegar a number of times each day for approximately three weeks. Later, a weak hydrogen peroxide solution was used.

When pain was intolerable and a tooth could not be saved, someone knowledgeable in pulling teeth instructed the "patient" to lie on the floor or a bed. The "dentist" propped open the mouth with a stick or similar object and held his knee against the chest as he pulled the offending tooth. A knife was used to cut about a quarter inch deep around the tooth. Tooth pullers sometimes slipped off a tooth, causing excruciating pain. When the tooth finally came out, the mouth was filled with salt to absorb any bleeding. Thankfully, my father did none of the above. However, his tooth-pullers, taken from the old family trunk and smelling of mothballs were bad enough.

Some children suggested another plan for extraction of their baby teeth. They tied one end of a string around the loose tooth and the other end to a doorknob. Then they waited for someone to open the door. I never actually saw this happen, but I heard that some children actually did it.

If a tooth was knocked out, we immediately tried to replace it using string to tie the lost tooth to the teeth on either side. Replaced teeth sometimes remained in position.

For problems with dentures, one can sprinkle some powdered slippery elm bark on gums to relieve discomfort and to make them adhere properly. If sores are on the gums, heap the powder on each side of the sore spot and eat whatever you like with no pain. Because slippery elm is also used for stomach ailments, there is no problem with swallowing it.

DEODORANTS – Underarm deodorants were not available to us in stores until perhaps the late 1930's. We sprayed a mixture of vinegar and water on the underarm area. Baking soda, which can be mixed with cornstarch, was also sprinkled in the area. Since aluminum, often found in deodorants, has been found in the brains of many deceased Alzheimer patients, I think we should use aluminum-free products for this purpose.

EYES – To remove puffiness and/or fine wrinkles under and around the eyes, apply sweet milk or vegetable shortening around the eyes before going to bed at night. For puffy eyes or dark circles, apply chilled tea bags or sliced chilled cucumbers to closed eyelids. Another remedy is to mix one-half tablespoon apple cider vinegar and one-tablespoon sweet oil and lightly rub the mixture around the eyes.

Today some swear by Preparation H. Carefully apply the product into the skin around the eyes being careful not to get it in the eyes. I tried it myself and had some success.

EYE COLOR - Mother, who grew up in these mountains, told us that jimson weed, which grew around the barn lot, would change eye color. She said she heard that crushing and putting the juice of jimson weed in blue eyes would turn the eyes so black that within 15 minutes your mother would not know you. This coloring was said to last 24 hours.

She never tried it. In fact, she was afraid to try it. And for good reason. With further research, it appears that the reason the eyes turn black is that jimson weed dilates the pupils. Consumption of any part of the jimson weed can be fatal.

36

EYE LASHES – I once used castor oil to make my eye lashes grow longer. It worked so well that the lashes rubbed the lenses of my glasses and made them sore. I soon stopped that treatment.

FOOT ODOR - Sprinkle shoes with baking soda to kill odor, or crumple pieces of newspaper and shove them into smelly footwear. Another possible solution is to soak one's feet in warm salt water.

FRECKLES – Many believed that you could remove freckles by applying stump water (found in the hollow of a stump) to them. In fact, I was told to try that remedy, but I never did. Freckles were removed with nitro-muriatic acid. A mixture of 30 drops in an ounce of water was applied and left on for some time.

HAIR – My father enjoyed telling us about a girl who watched two other girls who were combing their hair. He said he heard her say, "I don't see how you can stand to comb your hair every day. I just comb mine once a week, and it nearly kills me."

We liked to wash our hair in rainwater, which we carried to the kitchen sink from the cistern, a tank that collected rain as it came off the barn roof. Until we moved out of the Park, we usually used only homemade soap and vinegar for shampoos. Once we began buying shampoo (Selsun blue is the first commercial shampoo I remember), we were told to add one tablespoon apple cider vinegar to a 12-ounce bottle of shampoo and shake well.

The vinegar was supposed to thicken the shampoo so that you used less of it. When it is not possible to use water, rub hair well with cornmeal or cornstarch for a dry shampoo.

FEMININE HYGIENE - No feminine hygiene products were available. During their monthly periods, women added extra petticoats under their dresses to absorb the flow.

VARICOSE VEINS - Soak a piece of cheesecloth in witch hazel and wrap around the affected areas. A warm, moist application of bayberry is also supposed to reduce swelling associated with varicose veins. In addition, I have heard that Preparation H, which contains witch hazel and aloe, reduces spider veins.

WRINKLES - A somewhat primitive face-lift included tying some hairs together in the center top of the head and making them tighter every day. This technique was said to reduce wrinkles in the face and to stop coughs by raising the palate.

In the good old days, women once ironed their wrinkles. They used spoons and mugs of very hot and very cold water. Heating a spoon in the hot water, they held it against a crease or wrinkle. Then a cold spoon was held against the same wrinkle.

For facials, apply generous coats of beaten egg whites or oatmeal paste to wrinkles. Or, add apple cider vinegar to two cups of red clay. Beat the mixture to make a fine paste. After these mixtures dried, they were removed with cool water and mild soap.

Various forms of exercise using facial muscles were supposed to reduce facial wrinkles and flabbiness. Grimacing or pretending to hold a pencil in the mouth while writing words in the air were suggested as methods to improve the appearance of the face.

I apply pure apple cider vinegar at night when I think of it. I also believe frequently applying water to the face by wetting both hands and rubbing up and out can help a great deal.

A recent facial treatment requires a 2" chunk of fresh cucumber, which has been peeled and seeded. Add to this, one teaspoon lemon juice, one teaspoon witch hazel, one beaten egg white, two tablespoons of yogurt, and two tablespoons of non-fat powdered milk. Puree all in a blender. Apply the mixture to the face, and wait for 30 minutes before washing with warm water and mild soap.

A friend told of his 90-year-old grandmother, who looks to be about 40 years old. Every night, after going to bed, she takes both hands and pushes upward on her face.

DIGESTIVE ORGANS

Years ago, Annie Wallace, a fellow church member, and I experienced a food poisoning episode in which both of us were convinced that we were dying from heart attacks. We were at Camp Carson, a Baptist camp, about 60 miles north of Knoxville.

I lay there on a rough cot looking at the unfinished walls in our room, thinking about what an ugly place it was to die. I knew we were too far from Knoxville to consider getting medical help for my heart attack.

After a while, I decided I should tell Annie that I was dying. When I told her, her heels hit the floor. She said she was also dying and was wondering if there was any chance I could get her to Knoxville to a hospital.

When we looked at each other, some sanity kicked in. We realized that both of us would not be dying of a heart attack at the same time. We both started laughing until we hurt.

Finally, I realized I needed to go to the bathroom. When I opened the door, I discovered a line of perhaps 30 women extending up the hallway and around the corner waiting for the restrooms. We learned we were not alone with our "heart attacks." The entire group of perhaps 100 women was poisoned on potato salad.

Amazingly, Annie and I were the least sick of anyone. I have always attributed it to that good laugh we had.

I do not remember any cases of food poisoning at home, and digestive concerns were relatively rare. When they occurred, three remedies I remember were castor oil, baking soda, or turpentine.

ALCOHOL OR DRINKING PROBLEMS - We in these hills never heard of a social drinker or an alcoholic. We knew only of teetotalers (non-drinkers) or drunks. It was a given that the best way to hold your liquor was in the bottle. Over the years, I have collected some remedies related to the consumption of "demon drink," however.

It was suggested that an aid to stop drinking was to add baking soda to a glass of water and drink it when the urge to drink became too great. I am not sure of the amount of soda that was used, but I would not use more than one-half teaspoon.

A common remedy to prevent becoming intoxicated was to eat a big chunk of raw cabbage or coleslaw with vinegar before drinking alcohol. People also used to drink liquid antacids before parties to try to prevent getting drunk. Slowly sipping a glass of milk sprinkled with some nutmeg was thought to help neutralize or absorb some of the effects of alcohol.

If these preventative measures did not work, a remedy for hangovers was to eat ten strawberries or some pawpaws. Eating two tablespoons of honey every 20 minutes for one hour and repeating three, and then six hours later, was supposed to relieve symptoms of a hangover.

My daughter reported miraculous results from peach tree tea when a friend in college overindulged. Another suggestion was to drink a glass of sauerkraut juice. I think I would prefer living with the hangover.

APPENDICITIS - It saddens me to think how many lives were cut short, and how many people suffered because of lack of medical care and information. My great-grandfather, William Thomas Trentham, came in from the woodlands suffering with appendicitis. He died, leaving a pregnant wife and six children, of whom my grandfather, Robert Lee Trentham, age 12, was the oldest. My great-grandmother survived and lived some 30 more years. All their graves can be found in our old family cemetery just inside the Park entrance from Gatlinburg,

For appendicitis, old-timers applied a castor oil pack to the site for six hours without heat. Some believed echinacea was helpful.

CONSTIPATION - In my youth, many people used Black Drought, a well-known and well-advertised manufactured laxative. My father instructed an acquaintance to take as much loosely powdered Black Drought as would lie on a dime. When Dad saw the man a few days later, he asked if the Black Drought had worked for him. The man very shyly reported that he did not have a dime, but he had two nickels.

"Well? How was it?" asked my dad.
"I got my money's worth," the man replied.

Other remedies for constipation included:

- Boneset, an old remedy for constipation that apparently started with our Native American cousins. It was probably used in a tea.

- Drinking a tea made from peach tree leaves three times a day.

- Drinking a cup of hot water before breakfast. A doctor I know recently mentioned that his lifelong problem with constipation was solved by drinking two quarts of warm water before breakfast.

- Eating an apple at bedtime.

- Eating pawpaws each day.

CROHN'S DISEASE - After a family member with Crohn's disease had seen five doctors in New York without success, I recommended golden seal. The capsules can be purchased in health food stores today. The individual reported relief of her symptoms. I dug the roots of this plant, which we called *yellowroot*, for my mother when we lived in what is now the

Park. She used it for stomach distress. Other remedies for Crohn's disease are peach tree tea or peppermint tea.

DIARRHEA – If we needed treatment for diarrhea, our first thought was to reach for white sugar and turpentine. Most home-use turpentine bottles have a very small mouth. Holding a finger over the mouth, we let a drop of turpentine fall on a small amount of sugar one drop at a time. The sugar was used to allow us to divide the turpentine into smaller amounts. If the diarrhea was not too bad, a person started with one-half to one drop.

My dad used to say, "Too much turpentine can bind you over until next court." (Circuit rider judges came to the area infrequently.) This meant that it does its work too well if you get too much. We also drank black pepper in boiled milk or a mixture of charcoal from burnt toast scraped into a cup of hot water. Ugh!

We never used one other well-known combination of cinnamon and cayenne pepper. It was said that this remedy would tighten the bowels so quickly that it took longer to prepare it than for the tea to work. For sick stomach accompanied with diarrhea, some drank buttermilk with lots of black pepper. Apple cider vinegar mixed in drinking water is also said to help. Some suggest drinking apple cider vinegar 30 minutes before eating to prevent diarrhea when in a foreign country.

Other remedies include:

· Drink blackberry juice.

· Drink catnip tea or peppermint tea made from ½ to one teaspoon of the dried herb in warm water.

· An old Indian recipe was to drink a cup of warm milk to which a pinch of allspice was added.

· When my husband Ray and I lived in Texas as students just after World War II, Ray went to see a Dr. Newburn regarding a bad case of diarrhea. His prescription was to stop by the grocery en route home and buy the largest steak we could afford. The doctor said that eating the steak would give those worms something to eat on instead of his intestines. It worked.

FISHBONE - Eating a piece of bread can dislodge a fish bone in the throat. We also gargled with full strength lemon juice and then sipped the juice if needed. One time, my grandson got a bone stuck horizontally in his throat. We thought we had gotten it out, but a few days later, we looked again because the spot was still sore. After we had him gargle for about 30 minutes with lemon juice, the bone became soft enough to come up into his throat so we could remove it with tweezers.

FLATULENCE OR GAS DISCOMFORT – Before Gasex or Beano, mountain folk used a variety of remedies to reduce gas discomfort or flatulence. One remedy was to bring to a boil one cup of water mixed with two teaspoons allspice powder, and let the mixture steep 10 to 20 minutes. Drink up to three cups a day.

Another remedy is to take a mixture of one teaspoon grated fresh ginger pulp and one teaspoon lime juice immediately after eating, or drink peppermint or dill tea.

Vinegar poured on foods such as beans also reduces gas discomfort. To remove about 90% of the gas in beans, heat them to boiling in soda water. Rinse them and soak them all night in water. Then rinse the beans again before cooking.

When I worked at the hospital, we always made sure our patients ate applesauce if beans were served. However, we never ate applesauce with eggs. If you try it, you will know why.

We burned toast and used the carbon for gastric problems. Dr. Ralph Shilling, for whom I worked at the Gatlinburg Medical Center, wrote many prescriptions for charcoal tablets.

FOOD POISONING - We called it ptomaine poisoning. For this problem, some mountain families took one teaspoon of apple cider vinegar in six ounces of water every four minutes until the mixture was used up. Then they took one tablespoon of apple cider vinegar in six ounces of water every 20 minutes. Maybe the vinegar helps, because I have heard that the old greasy spoons (low quality restaurants) started serving pickles with sandwiches to keep customers from getting sick. Thus, the tradition of serving pickles with sandwiches.

Many years ago, my sister got food poisoning while atop Mt. LeConte in the Smokies. To treat her, someone poured high-proof whiskey in a cup and set it on fire. When it had burned, the residue was mixed with water for her to drink. I was not along on this trip, so I do not know the amounts used. However, I understand that it helped. Today, physicians may prescribe charcoal tablets, which absorb many times their weight in liquid or gases.

HEMORRHOIDS - were usually called piles. An old remedy used to relieve the symptoms was to peel a raw potato, shape it like a suppository, and insert it in the affected area as high as possible. Holding a compress saturated with lamp oil (kerosene) to the area provided relief from hemorrhoid discomfort, especially for irritated external hemorrhoids occurring after childbirth.

I understand that bayberry bark has been used as a remedy for hemorrhoids, but I am not sure if it is used as a tea or applied to the source of the problem.

HICCOUGHS - [HICCUPS] We mountain children "scared" the hiccups out of the victim. If there is no one around to scare you, chew a spoonful of mustard or some mustard seeds. A second remedy was to eat one teaspoon of sugar.

The old standby for hiccups was to slowly sip a glass of warm water mixed with one teaspoon of vinegar. It works better if you lean over and sip from the far side of the glass. Some left out the vinegar and simply sipped the water from the far side of a glass. I do not know that any of this really works, but it usually kept one busy until the hiccups went away on their own.

INDIGESTION AND BELLY (STOMACH) ACHE – In addition to the dose of castor oil our mother gave us if we complained, another remedy for dyspepsia was baking soda. When we were children, we put a small amount of bicarbonate of soda in a glass of water if we had "bellyache." Today, I know of a doctor who never travels without her baking soda.

My choice of remedies for gastric distress is golden seal, which we called yellowroot. I buy the capsules, open them, and put the contents in a glass of water for a very refreshing drink. Years ago, we dug the root and left it in water over night, and then drank the water. Old timers also relied on pawpaws for indigestion. Others liked to drink catnip, sage, or pennyroyal tea.

Mustard or mustard seed mixed with sweet oil (olive oil) helps with heartburn. Today, Dijon mustard is great. Another remedy is peach tree tea, which is described in more detail in the general remedies section at the end of the book. Sucking on a piece of ginger, eating two or three slices of a raw potato, or drinking a small amount of sauerkraut juice are also said to help.

Recently, when two neighbor women were complaining of heartburn, I told them to drink a small amount of apple cider vinegar mixed in water. Despite their disbelief, they agreed to try it. They later admitted that it helped them.

Preventative measures include taking a capsule of slippery elm powder before a meal or taking two or three chewable tablets of licorice daily on an empty stomach. Chamomile or evening primrose infusions are also said to be good for indigestion and gas discomfort.

OBESITY - The old, old cure for obesity and the secret to living as long as Methuselah, who the *Bible* says lived to be 969 years old, was simply chewing each mouthful of food until it became as water. Another strategy designed to slow down eating was to take a bite of food, and then lay down your fork until the bite was completely chewed and swallowed. Then pick up your fork again.

Other than increased exercise and reduced fat and carbohydrate diets doctors recommend for today, some substances have been suggested to help lose weight. They include honey, limejuice, ginger, cinnamon, black pepper, mint, and tomatoes. Some people have said that drinking a mixture of water, apple cider vinegar, and honey helps them to lose weight.

TOBACCO - Stop smoking mountain style. For a three-week period, take one-third teaspoon baking soda in water three times per day. During this time, eat primarily foods described as alkaline: apples, berries, carrots, celery, mushrooms, onions, peas, raisins, sweet potatoes, squash, and tomatoes. These foods are said to calm one down, as does the tobacco. No smoking or alcoholic beverages are allowed during this time.

VOMITING - Let an opened can of Coca-Cola stand until it goes flat (about 30 minutes.) Then drink it. Drinking it flat keeps the carbonation from further upsetting the stomach. Dr. Shilling prescribed Coke, but I do not recall that he said to let it go flat.

ULCERS - Until very recently, no one believed that bacteria caused peptic ulcers. Before the dramatic experiment in which a doctor drank a cup of bacteria to prove his theory, most people, including doctors, believed ulcers were caused primarily by stress. This was said to produce too much acid in the stomach. People with ulcers were cautioned to avoid stress.

One stomach ulcer treatment suggested eating servings of raw and cooked cabbage every day for three weeks. Some believe there is an enzyme in cabbage not yet identified that helps to cure ulcers. I remember that ulcer patients were often told to drink

51

milk and eat a bland diet. Pawpaws were also eaten to treat ulcers. Some used echinacea for this purpose.

GENERAL AILMENTS & AFFLICTIONS

We did not hear about many cures to diseases. When I was younger, a diagnosis of cancer nearly always meant death. There was no preventative care or effective treatment, and cancer was nearly always found long after the patient contracted the disease.

About 1958, when I had a skin cancer removed from my neck, I was sure I was dying. Because no one who had cancer ever survived it, I did not tell anyone about my condition. After a number of months, I realized I was probably going to live, and I went on with my life.

In 1969, I had a breast removed due to breast cancer. At that time, when you learned that someone had cancer, you just mentally buried him or her. A few months afterward, I called an acquaintance my husband and I knew. After I introduced myself, the man asked, "Are you sure this is Bonnie Myers?" I assured him that I was. When he asked a few more times, I realized that he thought I had died. I have often wished that I had been alert enough to ask, "Where do you think I am calling *from*."

Generalized ailments and chronic diseases are listed below with some of the remedies we and others believed would prevent or cure them.

CANCER - One of the more interesting cancer remedies I ran across involved Luella Pemberton's mother. Luella's mother washed clothes on a washboard to help her daughter go to college. In 1964, when she weighed 60 pounds, her doctors could do nothing else for her. They sent her home to die.

Luella was so distraught that she prayed day and night for a cure. When she began seeing dogwood blooms with her eyes open and closed, Luella decided this was a sign for a cure for her mother. She had never heard of anyone using dogwood to treat cancer, and she did not know if it was poisonous. However, she found a book in the Oak Ridge Library describing an Indian princess who was cured with dogwood tea. After initial reluctance, her mother drank the dogwood tea, and she fully recovered. Luella wrote about this experience in the Knoxville newspaper.

The tea was made by cutting pieces of a young dogwood tree into small pieces and exposing the interior of the wood. After cooking it in water in a stainless steel container for about six hours, she diluted it to taste and drank one-half cup four times a day.

Another cancer remedy used in this area is flaxseed oil eaten with cottage cheese. Recently, when the new cancer specialist in town prescribed some medication to try to stop some skin cancers on my face, he asked if I had used the medication he prescribed. I told him I did not want to pay the $100-$200 for the drug.

Instead, I told him I was using flaxseed oil with cottage cheese. Expecting him to be upset with me, I was amazed when he said, "Oh, that is good!" Maybe some doctors are open to non-prescription remedies.

I recall a newspaper article about a cancer forum in Louisiana about 1948 saying that wood pulp would cure cancer. Other home cancer remedies are listed below:

- Drinking teas made from red clover blooms or propolis mixed with brandy were said to cure stomach cancer. (Old time cures)

- Inhale apple brandy for the lungs.

- Eat at least three almonds every day to prevent cancer.

- In addition to possible benefits to vision, one raw carrot daily may prevent cancer. Brightly colored vegetables, said to contain carotenoids, are said to prevent cancers of lungs, colon, breast, uterus, and prostate.

I found it very interesting that one study indicated that wearing a bra more than 12 hours a day might increase the risk of breast cancer as much as 100 times. If bras affect breast cancer, I could easily have gone without all these years.

DIABETES – There was no insulin or Oranase available to treat diabetes, which we always called *sugar* diabetes, when I was growing up. We knew very little about the effects of diet and exercise on the disease.

55

My brother-in-law ate honey with his meals believing it could control his diabetes. Different remedies suggested eating honey straight from the jar, drinking three spoonfuls of honey in boiled water, or consuming honey mixed with two tablespoons of apple cider vinegar. Below are diabetes remedies I have collected.

- Some believe eating raw white potatoes or a mixture of flaxseed oil combined with cottage cheese, help to control blood sugar levels.

- Long before the arrival of the Europeans, Native Americans cultivated Jerusalem artichokes, which they called "sun roots." They were used as a treatment for diabetes.

- Mix one part bilberry tincture to one part bearberry tincture. Add 10 to 20 drops of this mixture to a glass of water between meals to control blood sugar. A tincture is a mixture of an herb and liquid, usually consumable alcohol.

- As much as 1/8 teaspoon of ground cinnamon is said to triple the effects of insulin and/or help control blood sugar. Cloves and sage are also supposed to be good for Type II Diabetes.

- People with diabetes were told to try fresh radishes, licorice, cinnamon, mint leaves, orange peels, or ginger root to ease a throbbing headache.

FATIGUE – (Remedies for increased energy) Walk barefoot on the grass if there is dew. If there is no dew, walk barefoot on the ground. Run for two minutes, or slap the inside of your elbows or the back of your knees.

Every morning, add two tablespoons of apple cider vinegar and one teaspoon honey to a cup of hot water and drink up. Some eat grapes, figs, or small amounts of bee pollen for increased energy.

When I was younger, if we felt unusually tired and sluggish for a period of time, we tested ourselves for thyroid function by painting a big spot of colored iodine somewhere on our bodies. If that spot was still colored the next morning, it meant we were OK. If there was little or no sign of the iodine, we knew our bodies needed iodine. My half-sister, Lillie Trentham Watson, had a goiter on her neck. She painted it with iodine every day for quite some time, and the goiter went away.

KIDNEY AND URINARY TROUBLE – My doctor told my mother and me that he would induce labor six weeks early for my first baby because of acute kidney infection or albumen poisoning. Out of earshot of the doctor, my mother said, "Humph, I'll take you home and make some punkin' (pumpkin) seed tea."

Bruising fresh pumpkin seeds, hull and all, she slowly brewed a pumpkin seed tea. Then, she made me drink this gosh-awful stuff. When I went back to the doctor the following week, the poison was gone. The doctor did not ask what I had done. Mother used the old field pumpkin seeds. The dark pumpkins we use for Halloween decorations today do not have good seeds. They are also not as good for eating. I ate many apples with the second and third pregnancies and had no kidney problems.

In addition to drinking pumpkin seed tea, other remedies for urinary problems include eating pumpkin seeds or drinking large amounts of cinnamon tea or cranberry juice.

Another common remedy was to boil the root of queen of the meadow. Drink a cup or more of this tea every four hours for two days. My father told my brother-in-law that one could drink it and piss over a ten-rail fence. My brother-in-law never mentioned if this was accurate. Others drank a tea made from pennyroyal or alfalfa for kidney problems.

I heard that for bladder infections outback hillbillies with no medication available found a slant board and propped it at least 30 degrees. Putting their feet at the top and their heads at the bottom, they massaged the bladder area for at least fifteen minutes while in this position. Apparently, this took the weight off the bladder area and allowed for better circulation.

LIVER – Until the 1960's, a highly advertised patent medicine, Carter's Little Liver Pills, was used for a variety of afflictions associated with the liver. After the U.S. government suggested that the pills had no effect on the liver, the name was changed to Carter's Little Pills. The pills soon dropped out of favor.

HEART, BLOOD AND BLEEDING

For many years, Smoky Mountain people have invoked the *Bible* verse found in Ezekiel 16:6 to stop bleeding. They substitute the victim's name in place of the word *thee.* "And when I passed by thee, and saw thee polluted in thine own blood, I said unto thee when thou wast in thy blood, Live: yea, I said unto thee when thou was in thy blood, Live." [King James Version]

My first experience using that scripture to stop bleeding occurred about 1950. It involved a patient at Blount Memorial Hospital who was dying from blood loss. His doctors could offer no further help. When my phone rang, the caller said a family member was bleeding to death. They had called every minister in the local telephone directory down to our name, Myers, to learn where to find the verse in the *Bible* that stops bleeding. I took the patient's name, the caller's name and phone number, and told her I would look it up in my Young's Analytical Concordance. I knew that *Bible* verse was the only verse having the word "blood" in it three times.

When I returned the call, the person who took the message immediately hung up. Then I started to worry. If they were depending on me, the patient was as good as dead. I watched the newspaper for days, and the patient's name never appeared in the obituary column.

An amazing instance in which this scripture was used occurred recently in Maryville, Tennessee. A very large man had an epileptic seizure and fell backward onto a showcase. He shattered the glass and suffered a number of severe cuts on his head. While the ambulance was en route to a hospital, someone asked for a *Bible* and read Ezekiel 16:6. According to the report, the bleeding had almost stopped by the time the ambulance arrived at the hospital.

ANEMIA - We knew that iron was necessary for health, but I am not sure that when I was a child, we understood what iron did for us. We got our iron from rusty nails and cooking in an iron skillet. Before the advent of vitamin tablets, some mountain folk actually put rusty nails in water to obtain iron.

We were told that beer, wine, and other alcoholic beverages depleted the body of iron, which made anemia worse. We believed eating pawpaws helped with anemia. Today, we can drink ginseng tea or eat raw spinach.

BLEEDING – In addition to using the *Bible* verse for very serious bleeding, a very old remedy was to cover an open wound with cobwebs and brown sugar pressed together like lint. Another was to apply lampblack, sometimes mixed with lard. I do not remember that we ever used either of these remedies at our house.

BLOOD CLOTTING - We knew that cinnamon made pumpkin pies taste great, but we did not realize that it is also supposed to be a great blood thinner. We have heard that cloves may be a better blood thinner than aspirin. Chili peppers and sassafras tea are also suggested.

BLOOD POISONING - Before the days of antibiotics or tetanus shots, a woman came to our home with red streaks going up the veins in her badly swollen arm. We called it blood poisoning.

My father mixed equal parts of sulfur, gunpowder, and alum. The woman took orally what would lie on a dime. Then, my father added vinegar to the mixture and applied it in a poultice to her arm. Much improved, she went home within three days.

BLOOD – Burdock and raw sauerkraut were both said to be great blood purifiers, used to remove toxins from the blood.

HEART PROBLEMS - If a person had poor circulation and swelling of ankles and legs due to heart problems, is was called dropsy. Various remedies were suggested for heart problems. One was to take two teaspoons of honey each day. Another was to eat a lot of garlic or ginger. Bayberry bark used in a tea was also supposed to be good for circulation.

For a fast heartbeat, we heard that immersing the nose and/or the head in cold water slows down fast heartbeats. (I wonder if an ice pack would help just as much.)

HIGH BLOOD PRESSURE – Possibly the best know home remedy for high blood pressure is garlic. Other remedies for high blood pressure are:

- Eat celery or take celery seeds steeped in a tea.

- Some people eat molasses or pawpaws.

- Another suggested remedy is a tea made of evening primrose.

- Chives, once thought to drive away evil spirits and disease, have also been used to lower blood pressure.

NOSE BLEEDING - Many youngsters had nosebleeds years ago. I recall when I had nosebleeds, I would pinch my nostrils shut, or we burned leather and inhaled the fumes. Others rolled up a piece of brown paper bag and put the roll between their teeth and upper lip to stop nosebleed.

Another remedy called for covering a banana peel (pawpaw) and some corn silk with water in a pan. After bringing it to a boil, remove from the heat, strain, and then cool the liquid before drinking it.

INFECTIOUS DISEASES & SANITATION

When I was about eight or nine years old, I remember that all my family except for me were in bed with flu. With milking and feeding the cows and caring for the mules, pigs and chickens, I had a lot of responsibility. Since my family had nothing to eat, I tried to make some biscuits for them. Because I did not know to add more dry flour to make biscuits smooth, I produced a gooey sticky mess. The outside of the biscuits looked something like porcupine quills sticking straight up.

My brother Harmon was the first to see them. He grabbed the pan and raced all over the house to show everyone those awful-looking biscuits. I do not recall if anyone ate any of the biscuits, but I think I developed a life-long aversion to cooking after that.

Soon after my attempt to make biscuits, Marjorie Chalmers, the nurse from the Pi Beta Phi School in Gatlinburg, came to check on us. When I leaned against the bed where she was examining my sister Kate, she pushed me away saying, "Don't touch her bed." Innocent like, I said, "Why, I sleep with her."

The nurse made a big fuss and asked my mother if she had another place for me to sleep. Because there were so many of us children, we slept two to a bed. After the nurse left, I did not give it another thought. I continued sleeping in the bed with my sister and also did not get flu.

We were aware that diseases were contagious, but we were not always sure how to prevent the spread of disease or infection. I have listed below some of our sanitation measures, infectious diseases of concern to us, and some of our treatments.

CHICKEN POX – When a child contracted chicken pox, we did very little except to keep a him or her comfortable possibly giving sponge baths with cool water. Some suggested a tea of echinacea or catnip. I did not know of any cases of adult chicken pox.

DECONTAMINATION – To disinfect a room, old-timers heated a shovel quite hot and slowly poured vinegar over it. At the same time, they would open the windows. I suppose opening the windows let out the odor of vinegar and may have taken some of the germs with it. Some believed that placing a piece of cut onion in the room would absorb germs where someone was sick. For this reason, some would place a piece of onion under the bed of a sick person.

DIPHTHERIA – Because of childhood inoculations in the U.S., we rarely hear of diphtheria today. When I was a child, it was a devastating disease, killing many children and adults. Kerosene, better known then as coal oil or lamp oil, was the only folk remedy early people had. The treatment was to dip a clean white cloth in pure kerosene and swab the patient's throat. Adults swallowed as much as a tablespoon of the oil. This caused one to vomit the deadly mucus. Primitive as it was, it was credited with saving lives. Another suggested remedy was propolis. I am not sure how it was used. I suppose the patient chewed it.

HEPATITIS – Milk thistle was used to treat hepatitis and cirrhosis of the liver. I never learned how it was used.

MEASLES – Unlike the situation in which my sister Gladys nearly died of measles, most cases of measles are relatively mild. The patient was put to bed and given mainly liquids. Sometimes strong teas were given to help break out the rash that goes with the disease. In his book, Dr. Pierce suggested a daily bath in tepid water or drinking warm tea from plants, such as burdock to make the patient perspire. Echinacea was also used to treat the symptoms of measles.

SANITATION - RESTROOMS - Our toilet facilities were the wooden outhouses back of the house. When we lived in the Park, my half-brother had a freestanding "dark room" where he developed film. In fact, in 1913, he made what was perhaps the first photograph of Gatlinburg, a copy of which I have today. We turned his dark room into a rather luxurious toilet facility. It had seats for three adults and one child, and it was fur-lined in the wintertime. My sister claims there was a heater there, but I do not recall that.

During the summer, tree leaves or corncobs were usually used for toilet paper. My husband Ray claimed he once mistakenly used poison ivy leaves for this purpose. There were both white and red corncobs. The joke was that you used a red corncob first. Then you used a white cob to see if you needed to use another red cob. The cobs were rough.

We also used the pages from catalogs, such as the one from Sears & Roebuck. I do not remember that they were glossy back then. We wrinkled them up for better traction. In winter, when no leaves were available, strips of newspaper or washable rags were used. We subscribed to the Knoxville Journal.

TYPHOID – Because many genuinely believed it was best to starve a fever, patients with an elevated temperature received only liquids. My mother-in-law, Ida Jane Headrick Myers, said she lost a lot of weight when she contracted typhoid fever in the late 1920's. She said the excess weight she carried for the rest of her life was a result of regaining that weight (and more) after the fever. I do not know what Ida would have been given as a treatment. Dr. Pierce's remedy was tepid tub baths every three hours to reduce the fever.

It was said that typhoid could be cured by a tea made of boneset. Some doctors used Echinacea.

WATER – We heard that the way to determine if a source of water was safe to drink was to put one cup of water in a clean jar and add two tablespoons of sugar. Tighten the lid, and place the jar in a warm lighted room. If the water remained clear after 9 days, we were told it was safe to use. (I doubt this would meet today's standards.)

When I was a child, we children declared that if water flowed over seven rocks, it was safe to drink. I am sure the good Lord was watching over us. However, we were never aware of any problems with contaminated drinking water.

We carried water from the springhouse for drinking and cooking. We heated it on the wood-burning cook stove for bathing and dishwashing. When we moved to Pigeon Forge, a pitcher pump in a well furnished cooking and bath water. I remember one very cold day, my wet hand stuck to the pump. Family members had to pour very warm water on my hand to release me.

WHOOPING COUGH – (Pertussis) A number of remedies were used to treat whooping cough. In addition to his Golden Medical Discovery, Dr. Pierce said that Belladonna (deadly nightshade), a narcotic, was an excellent treatment. In our area, we used remedies such as raw garlic, evening primrose, or black

67

cohosh, the herb used for many female problems. [Cohosh is also spelled *cohash* and pronounced differently.] Some apparently used brown sugar mixed with kerosene. I hear this may actually have been ingested, but I would not try it myself.

INJURIES & FIRST AID

Because the *Bible* said Sunday was the day of rest, we only accomplished the essentials on that day. We fed the animals and milked the cows, but we engaged in no other labor except warming the food, which Mother cooked the day before.

On Sunday afternoon after we went to church, Mother always visited neighbors. One Sunday afternoon, when I was about seven or eight years old, as my mother was leaving to visit neighbors, she said to my siblings and me, "Now, don't ride that old mule." We, of course, watched until she got out of sight and immediately ran to find the mule. My sister Gladys sat in the saddle holding Sam, who is younger than I, in front of her. They rode for some distance, and it was clear they were not going to let me ride. After I told them I would tell Mother and threatened to make the mule run with them, they stopped and let me get on the back of the mule behind the saddle and the two of them.

We had hardly gone fifteen feet when I fell off and broke my right arm above and below the elbow and fractured the socket. Even today, you can see the effects of that fall. Without my mother's warning, we probably would never have thought of riding the mule.

Dad and my half-brother, attempted to set the bone for me. They put me between the bedroom wall and the head of a four-poster bed. The two of them stood in front of the bed board and pulled on my arm. Amid my screams and crying, they continued to try to set my arm. When that did not work, I saw a doctor, who put a cast on my arm. Doctors told me later that fluid leaked out of my elbow, which caused my arm to grow out of line.

The injury made playing the piano and typing a little difficult over the years, but I have used it to hit a mean baseball and to become the county champion volleyball server. I also made the high school basketball team, but my mother refused to allow me to wear the basketball bloomers in order to play. Those bloomers were full-cut and came down to my knees, but most church-going people believed that it was sinful for females to wear pants. Mother should see what I wear today. Below, I have included information about treatments I have collected for injuries.

BANDAGES – We were unable to buy band-aids, sterile gauze, and tape early on. For bandages, we used bed sheets or pillowcases torn into strips. With no tape, we tore strings from sheets to hold bandages in place.

BROKEN BONES – When a bone was broken, someone tried to set it in ways similar to what I described earlier. To hold the bone in place, a cast was necessary. Most often, our homemade casts were made of red clay mixed with water. The clay mixture was plastered around splints placed on each side of the broken bone and allowed to dry. A clay cast was as firm as the ones later formed in doctors' offices.

An interesting treatment for a broken hand was to place a good-sized ball of yarn in the palm of the hand and close the fingers around it. Then bandages were wrapped around the hand.

We did not have sterile cotton balls and bandages back then. When a person broke his or her nose, someone rolled up lint balls of sufficient size to fit each nostril and pressed the lint as far back in the nostril as possible. This was supposed to hold the broken fragments in place. These balls of lent were found under beds and saved for this purpose.

CUTS – We usually used turpentine or kerosene (coal oil) to sterilize and heal cuts. Deep flesh wounds were filled with the oil, and they usually healed very well. Some people in this area today keep a clean jar of kerosene close by to apply to puncture wounds. When it became available, we used iodine for puncture wounds. We also used alcohol to clean wounds. Both of these really stung when applied to a cut.

LIGHTNING – We were told that we should dash cold water over the chest or abdomen and apply hot bottles of water to the feet if someone were struck by lightning. Another suggestion was to apply a mustard plaster to the heart, hold ammonia briefly under the nostrils, or give whiskey if a person could drink it.

71

POISONS – A family secret we did not tell our children for many years was that one of my great grandfathers used a deadly rat poison for nefarious purposes. He and his female housekeeper decided to give it to my great-grandmother to get rid of her. As the wife ate lunch, she noticed the two of them kept suggesting that she drink some water. I believe the water was supposed to activate the rat poison. She realized they had poisoned her. As she ran out of the house toward her parents' house, she was quoted as saying, "You old b…. You poisoned me."

Her parents' house must have been about two miles away. Oddly, the husband and housekeeper never caught up with her, and she arrived at her parents' house. She remained with them for about two years before she died from the effects of the poison.

This man is buried in a cemetery on Ski Mountain Road in Gatlinburg. It is on the right side of the road a short distance after one crosses the river bridge going toward the lodge. His tombstone is inscribed *Richard Reagan*. When I visited the cemetery, I failed to look for his wife's grave. I do not know if she was buried in the same cemetery as he was.

Various remedies were suggested to counteract poisons. For ingested poisons, an emetic (something to induce vomiting) was prescribed. I have listed some of those remedies below.

· Ammonia (inhaled) - inhale vapors of vinegar.

72

- Arsenic - tickle the throat to induce vomiting. Give oils, eggs, fats, sweet milk, or starch.

- Alcohol – (poisoning) After administering an emetic of salt and water, give the victim strong coffee, and dash cold water all over his or her body.

- Lye – Emetics of lemon juice, oils, fats, butter, or vinegar and water were suggested back then. However, the protocol today is to avoid inducing vomiting due to the corrosive effects of lye. Another remedy was to give the victim flaxseed tea.

- Tobacco - Promote vomiting by giving castor oil or holding ammonia to the nose. In some cases, parents believed it was best to let a child suffer a good dose of sickness from smoking cigarettes to prevent them from taking up the habit when they were older. In fact, one of my family members deliberately gave his sons a large amount of strong cigarettes in order to make them sick. They never smoked again. That would probably be frowned on today.

REMOVE A SPLINTER - A bread and milk poultice was bandaged on the skin to bring out a splinter. Another remedy was to bind a piece of raw onion over the splinter. Today a suggestion is to cover the skin with Elmer's glue-all, wait for it to dry, and peel it off the skin.

TETANUS – When I was a child, we eagerly waited for the end of May so that we could go barefoot for the summer. At least once each summer, one of us children stepped on a rusty nail. This occurred before tetanus shots were available. We most often bruised peach leaves and bound them on the site. We had no fear of lockjaw. When I repeated this remedy to Dr. Joe Henderson,

73

our family doctor when our children were young, he said the good Lord was definitely watching over us.

WOUNDS – As mentioned before, cobwebs (spider webs) were spread over open wounds to stop bleeding, but I do not recall my parents ever using cobwebs this way. Kerosene was widely used to treat wounds. In fact, old timers can tell you amazing stories of how kerosene was the only treatment for puncture wounds.

Other remedies for wounds include:

- For open wounds, disinfect with propolis, sugar or kerosene.
- Slippery elm powder, used as a poultice, has been used with good results to draw out infection. Mix with water or with Vaseline for longer-lasting poultices.
- Sage leaves were sometimes bound on wounds to speed healing.
- During wartime, they used vinegar to disinfect wounds. For eye infections, they diluted the vinegar.
- During World War II, when supplies were late or missing, they put cloves of raw garlic on the edges of a wound to promote healing.

MENTAL CONCERNS, HEADACHES & SLEEP ISSUES

I often think of how my late husband Ray T. experienced the hell of the South Pacific at Guadalcanal and Bougainville. He was one of five from his company (M, 182nd Infantry) who survived. He said there were times when he just wanted to stand up and let the enemy kill him.

His malaria and debilitating fungus infection called jungle rot became so bad that he was eventually shipped home. Ray lost 65 pounds. He wandered alone in the jungle at Bougainville for 28 days with only wild onions and cocoanuts to eat. Until he happened to hear another member of his company interviewed on radio a few months after his return, he thought he was the only survivor from his company.

The soldiers understood that if they heard a bomb whistling as it came in their direction, it had their name on it. Ray and a buddy were sitting on the bank of the Lunga River when they heard that whistle. Clawing and scratching at the steep embankment behind them, they could not get out of the way. The bomb hit and splashed water on them. It was a dud!

He spent nine months in military hospitals. For several months after he returned home, he was not able to look directly at me or our infant son, Don. It appeared that he was looking through us into the distance. Until his death in 1976, he continued to experience nightmares in which the enemy was capturing him. I tried to awaken him by touching him only one time. He awoke before he hurt me, and he paced the floor for the rest of the night. After that, he asked me never to touch him when he was having a nightmare.

Ray returned from World War II with no understanding of post-traumatic stress disorder. He never would have considered psychotherapy even if it had been available. At that time, only the "very weak" thought about receiving professional help.

We generally attributed mental illness to character traits or personal failings. Someone who acted oddly was sometimes described as "a mite quare." People who suffered from depression or compulsive behavior tried to keep it to themselves. As in much of America at that time, if people suffered from depression, phobias or perhaps obsessive-compulsive disorders, they were just considered odd or weak. We usually did not recognize disorders associated with the brain or nervous system as treatable. Some of our opinions and treatments are listed below.

ANGER – In my family, we rarely talked about emotions or confronted anger. If we became angry with one another, one of us left the room or the house until we were no longer angry. Or, Ray always tried to make me laugh. It seemed to work. We were happily married for nearly 36 years.

Mountain wisdom says to look to the earth to release anger. Walk barefoot on the ground. Listen to the sounds of rushing waters, singing birds, or wind rustling through the leaves. Screaming when alone, pounding a pillow, or breaking dishes may also help. Today, maybe it is better to discuss it calmly.

DEPRESSION – Many used the term "out of heart" to describe what we would call depression today. We did not recognize this as a medical condition. Some suggested pawpaws as a treatment.

EPILEPSY - Epilepsy was called the *falling sickness* or having *fits*. Mountain folk drank a tea made from the root of the male peony plant. The tea was steeped for twenty-four hours, strained, and consumed over a period of several days. To cure young children, the peony root was hung around the neck of the child. I doubt the FDA would approve our remedy.

Another mountain remedy was made from the root, seeds, and leaves of parsley mixed with anise and caraway. These ingredients were steeped in white wine until one-third of the liquid evaporated. Patients drank four ounces morning and evening. They were supposed to refrain from drinking any other beverage for three hours afterward.

FAINTING – Women seemed much more prone to fainting back then. If a woman fainted because of female conditions, old-timers sometimes said she had "the vapors." In Victorian times, people had fainting couches. We could not afford this luxury.

Fainting often occurred at funerals, where we heard there were sometimes hired mourners or "professional fainters." As an adult and the wife of the minister, I was always armed with vials of smelling salts, which funeral directors supplied for fainters. The vials were crushed by hand and had a very strong ammonia odor. One whiff usually brought the fainter around. I believe these vials put a stop to our "professional fainters."

Ray conducted many funerals. One woman fainted at every funeral she attended. Finally, disgusted with this exhibition, he grabbed the woman up from the floor without a word, carried her outside, sat her down on the church steps, yanked her dress down over her knees, and left her sitting there. I do not believe she ever fainted in one of his funeral services again.

If mountain folk became faint from fieldwork in the sun, and they became pale around the eyes and mouth, they were described as being "white-eyed." We never hear this expression today. Then again, perhaps we do not work that hard anymore. To prevent this condition, one can put a big green leaf in your hat while working outside in hot weather.

FEEBLE-MINDEDNESS – Today, we would say an individual is mentally challenged or slow. We used the term feeble-minded. Ben Trentham, my grandfather's brother, had an extremely bad case of measles. Because sick folk were not allowed to eat any food, Ben sneaked out at night and ate lots of green apples. Whether it was the apples or his illness, Ben spent the rest of his life as simple-minded or feeble-minded. Both terms were used.

There were a number of interesting stories involving Ben. Before the days of refrigerators, Ben once helped himself to the milk in a neighbor family's springhouse. When the neighbor asked Ben if he had taken the family's milk, his reply was, "If I did, I didn't have any cornbread to go with it." What could be said to that?

My dad's favorite story about Ben was the time Ben had annoyed my father to his breaking point. Dad threatened him and said, "Ben, if you don't stop that, I'm going to go get my gun and shoot you."

With that, Dad went into the house, forgetting all about Ben. After quite some time Ben, still waiting outside, called out, "Noah, if you don't come on and shoot me, I am going to leave!"

Local church-going people walked to Evans Chapel Church, located behind where the Great Smoky Mountains National Park headquarters of today. Ben made his toilet stops along the main road by just pulling his cap down over his eyes. Apparently, he believed that if he could not see others, they could not see him.

There was no treatment or training available for those in Ben's condition. Parents or siblings generally cared for them. If they were too hard to handle, they were placed in the Knoxville "insane asylum" known as Lyons View.

GROUCHINESS – I do not remember anyone so afflicted, but violet blossom tea was supposed to be good for that condition. We never believed anything would really help grouchiness.

HEADACHES - Ray had migraine headaches, which began when he was a young child. He often poured Stanback headache powders straight out of a package into his upturned mouth. I do not remember that he even drank water with the powders.

Bess Trentham, wife of my half-brother Mack, would tie a white rag around her head. I do not know if it really helped, but she seemed to think it did. Other headache remedies include:

· Inhale the steam of hot water to which a dash of vinegar is added. This is supposed to relieve headaches in 20 minutes.

· Apply red pepper to the forehead.

· Chew the leaves of feverfew. However, this can cause irritation of lips and tongue.

- Drink a tea of echinacea. Some drank a tea of pennyroyal. However, it has risks described more fully in the last section of the book.

- Modern remedies include efforts to reduce the blood flow in the brain. This is accomplished by swinging the arms vigorously or imagining that the sun or a fire is warming ones hands.

- Massage the area between the thumb and index finger vigorously for 3-4 minutes.

HYPOCHONDRIACS - MOUNTAIN STYLE - A very strange malady seemed to afflict a few mountain women. For some unexplained reason, they spent most of their lives in bed. We spoke of them as being "hippoed." This was possibly a corruption of the word *hypochondria*. It seemed to everyone that these women were not really sick.

I recall a hippoed mother and daughter coming to our house to visit when I was young. The woman was the wife of our minister at the time. As they came through the front door, the mother said to her daughter, "I'll take the bed, and you can take the couch." She went to my parents' bedroom and lay on their bed while the daughter stretched out on our couch. The husband visited with us. Reportedly, when the husband died, the woman heard noises - possibly her husband. Because of her "condition," she did not get out of her bed to investigate.

I recall one instance in which a family member was being buried, and someone returned home unexpectedly. This unexpected visit required the "hippoed" woman to jump into bed still wearing her shoes. Another time, a family member came home unexpectedly, and this "patient" was in the back field digging potatoes.

I cannot imagine why they chose to spend their lives in bed sneaking out when no one was around. I never heard of a man being "stricken" with this strange malady. Maybe they got tired of the hard work and used this to get the family to help with all the chores. Maybe there was really something wrong.

INSOMNIA - Had we ever heard the word *insomnia*, we probably would not have known what it meant. Few in our day had to be rocked to sleep. Working so hard to complete all the chores required to be able to eat and stay comfortable was a full time job. It is likely most everyone fell into bed exhausted at the end of the day.

Our only suggestion for sleep problems was to count sheep or drink some milk warmed to body temperature. Another suggestion was to add three teaspoons of apple cider vinegar to one cup of honey. Keep this mixture refrigerated, and take one teaspoon 30 minutes before bedtime. Chamomile tea is also supposed to be very good to help someone sleep.

MENTAL ILLNESS – Just as care for the feeble-minded was lacking, care for those we would call mentally ill was inferior. Someone who was mentally ill might be called a knucklehead, loony, or off his rocker. When I was quite young, a neighbor was declared mentally ill early in her life. This child somehow indicated that wild animals might live under their house, and she did so much swinging on their front porch that her feet wore a spot in the floor under the swing. Her family judged from her actions that she was insane, and that was that. So, she was sent to Lyons View in Knoxville.

Recently, my sister Gladys, and I went to Lyons View to visit her after she had been committed for some 60 years. Instead of being insane, we learned that her life-long problem was the fact that she was completely deaf.

I was amazed that she had learned to read and write so well under those circumstances. She was able to communicate by writing, and she appeared quite intelligent. What a shame she spent her life that way. No one knew a young person could be deaf.

One member of the family made very cruel comments to her young niece and nephew about how they were related to someone who was crazy. When I learned she was actually deaf, I did not let my shirttail touch my backside until I wrote those kids telling them what we had learned about their aunt.

SENILITY – I do not recall any elderly person during my early years who seemed to have a memory problem. The subject was never mentioned.

Old timers believed apple cider vinegar was a "cure-all." They believed in order to stay healthy and alert into old age one should combine one teaspoon of vinegar and one teaspoon of honey in a full glass of water and drink this mixture 1/2 hour before each meal. This was also supposed to improve memory. Another remedy was ginseng- either chewed or drunk in a tea.

I believe there is something in our modern lifestyle that is causing so much Alzheimer's disease. Because high levels of aluminum and zinc have been found in the brain tissue of people with Alzheimer's, it seems that we should avoid aluminum by checking contents of deodorants and not cooking in aluminum pots and pans. I also believe talking about memory problems so much contributes to the problem.

STRESS – When I was younger, we said that a person experiencing stress had a case of "nerves." Ginseng is said to help people coping with stress and working too hard stay mentally alert. Mountain folk carried ginseng roots in their pockets. When beginning to feel tired, they would put a root in their mouths to give them physical and mental energy. Another remedy for nerves, sometimes suggested, was to eat pawpaws.

PESTS: INSECTS, SNAKES, AND OTHER VERMIN

With panthers, bears, wildcats, snakes, mosquitoes, ticks, lice, and others, we had to contend with many pests. Although there were occasional bears in the area, I do not remember one ever coming on our property. However, I am quite sure I heard a panther yell just across the fence from me when I lived in the Park.

Snakes were our most constant and worrisome pests. In our family, because of snakes and other large animals, my Mother always took her old faithful shotgun when we went berry picking. She sometimes had the opportunity to use it on the snakes. I remember when Sam and I had found some luscious blackberries on a small bush. Both of us were rushing to get our part of those beautiful berries. After quite some time picking, we saw movement within inches of berries we were picking. In horror, we realized the movement was the tail of a copperhead snake lying stretched out on the limb holding all our berries.

Our screams that a copperhead was in a tree were ignored because "copperheads do not climb trees." Mother came with her shotgun and proved that two small children knew a copperhead when we saw one.

The story goes that around 1930, when my husband Ray was a child, he and his brothers were helping to build a swimming pool in Wears Valley. A big rock rolled onto his left forefinger and crushed everything below the top of the nail. While en route to Sevierville to see a doctor, his father, Bruce, spied a rattlesnake beside the road. Apparently more concerned with the snake than with his child's pain, Bruce stopped the buggy, got out, and shot the rattlesnake. Regarding the loss of his fingertip, Ray told our children that he was picking his nose, and a booger bit it off. They said they believed him until they were old enough to know better.

Every time Ray stepped out of the house, he said his mother always said, "Now, be careful of snakes." For that reason, he was always deathly afraid of them. Snakes were not our only concern, however. Below I have listed how we dealt with various pests.

ANTS - To get rid of ants, place red or black pepper, ground cloves, lemon juice, or white vinegar in their path. Mix equal parts powdered sugar and borax with water to make a paste. When ants eat this, they die. When ants eat their fallen comrades, those also die. Eventually this kills the whole colony. To trap ants, make a paste of one-third cup molasses, six tablespoons sugar, and six tablespoons dry yeast. Place the mixture on cardboard in an area where ants travel.

To deter ants, place cucumber peels in spots they are likely to go. Ants will also not cross a chalk line. Rub chalk on the threshold of the door. I tried it and found that it worked for me. Ants go crazy and run in circles trying to avoid it.

BEDBUGS – I recently read that bedbugs are making a comeback, even in fine homes and hotels. The one time we discovered bedbugs at our house, our solution was to take the headboards, footboards and side rails outside and treat them with kerosene. That was the last of them. Others said that burning sulfur in a closed room would eliminate the creatures.

We had no idea where the insects came from or how they got into our house. Perhaps an overnight guest brought them in their luggage. Before all the hotels were built in Gatlinburg and Pigeon Forge, if anyone asked to spend the night at someone's house, it was expected that we would welcome them and provide them with dinner and breakfast, even if they were strangers. This often happened at our house, and we never charged them a penny.

CHIGGERS (RED BUGS) - To avoid getting chiggers, we rubbed pennyroyal weed on our wrists and ankles before picking berries. Kerosene put on the cuff of pants or soles of the shoes was also considered a deterrent.

A quick bath or a swim in our swimming hole after picking berries generally washed off chiggers. Before nail polish was available to paint on chigger bites, we smeared imbedded chiggers with lard mixed with lots of salt. This mixture killed them, but the itch remained.

INSECT BITES - If an insect bit us when we were out in the fields, we gathered the leaves of seven weeds, crushed them, and rubbed the juice on the bite. If at home, we made a paste of either baking soda or Epsom salts mixed with water to rub on insect bites. Today, ammonia is used as an excellent remedy for most insect bites. It is sold in pharmacies under a variety of names.

For bee or hornet stings, first scrape out the stinger, if any, being careful not to squeeze it. A "spat of backer" (spit of tobacco juice) is said to be good for bee stings. I was recently talking with a friend who told about his first bee sting. He said his grandfather grabbed a chew of tobacco out of his mouth and said, "Here, put this on the bit!" He was so shocked that when his sting was better, he did not know if it was the tobacco or the shock that helped.

Howard Kerr, my beekeeper friend, said that those who rob beehives carry a box of salt with them. When they are stung, they just spit into their hands and then pour the salt in the spit to make a paste to put on the site of the sting. He said it was the best remedy ever. Others apply melaleuca oil (tea tree), meat tenderizer, aspirin, or the inside of a pawpaw or banana peel. Also, rub on ragweed, baking soda, or raw onion.

For mosquito bites, a number of ingredients were applied: wet tobacco or snuff, wet soap, vinegar, lemon juice, the inside of a pawpaw peel, or mud. I have also heard that one can spray with WD-40 for instant relief. It is also said to work for fire ant bites.

When an insect got into an ear, they poured a small amount of sweet oil (olive oil) into the ear to float it out. On rare occasion, someone gets a bee sting inside their mouth when eating apples or grapes. Mix two teaspoons of salt in water and continue gargling. It helps to keep the area from swelling. I have heard that one should swirl an open can or drink before drinking to make sure no insects are in it.

To prevent insect bites or stings, wear drab colors. It is also said that one should not wear blue. Bright clothing, perfume, and cologne attract insects. To prevent mosquito bites, mountaineers put oil of cloves mixed with Vaseline on hands and face and then sprinkled oil of cloves on their clothing. If one can stand the smell, rub garlic over the exposed skin. Rubbing with fresh parsley or pennyroyal sometimes helps also. Today, many swear by Avon Skin-So-Soft.

LICE – (HEAD AND BODY) My family never had any encounters with them to my knowledge. We heard that kerosene could be used to get rid of them. A common belief was that a walk in the rain on the first day of May would rid you of lice. I do not know what one did if he or she developed a case of lice at some other time of the year.

If a person caught head lice, a common treatment was to rinse with kerosene, which was left on the head for a short time before it was washed out. This treatment was repeated as necessary. The treatment worked, but kerosene has a strong, offensive odor that lingers everywhere. Some used yellow oxide of mercury ointment. I do not know how it was used, but further investigation indicated it is best to avoid it because of concerns about mercury poisoning. Another remedy was to shampoo with coal tar soap.

PIN WORMS - Mountain people believed that when the area around the mouth was whiter than the surrounding skin, the person had worms. Some ate only raw cabbage and drank tea three times a day to get rid of them. Eating rhubarb is also supposed to eliminate worms.

POISON IVY – We always remembered, "Leaves of three; let it be!" However, when I come in contact with poison ivy, I use a remedy, which has worked very well for me. It must be used at the first sign of allergic reaction. To relieve the itch, mix equal parts of salt and apple cider vinegar. Heat the mixture as warm as

90

can be tolerated and apply it to the skin with a clean cloth. In addition to a call from a chiropractor from Knoxville, I have had calls from New York, North Carolina, and New Jersey asking for my salt and vinegar cure.

Howard Kerr tells of a miraculous poison ivy treatment. He rubbed the leaves of the horehound weed on the site and got immediate relief. Tomato juice is also supposed to be good.

Gene LeQuire once said "Do not use boiled poke root juice for poison ivy or itch unless your are planning to run in a marathon and want to win first place!" Apparently, pokeroot and echinacea have also been used to treat poison ivy as well.

POISON OAK - The root of the bloodroot plant has been used to treat poison oak. Rub on the skin either the sap from a freshly broken root or a tincture made by soaking several cut roots in alcohol. Never take bloodroot internally.

RATS, MICE - We always kept a cat, which took care of any mice that might find their way to our house. However, wild mint planted around a house was supposed to keep mice and rats out.

RINGWORM – The most common mountain remedy was to apply the juice of black walnut hulls. Years ago, my son, Don, picked up ringworm. We thought he got it in a barbershop. A woman cured it using a piece of notebook paper rolled into a cone shape. She burned the paper and let the residue, a yellow oil, drop onto a plate. She then applied the oil to his head. The treatment stung so that he danced around for a while, but this remedy cured him.

An old mountain woman, who was known as a wizard, had a cure for everything. She rubbed ringworm with the inside of a cut green persimmon. This treatment also burned badly, but I hear the ringworm was cured. Another suggested remedy was simply to apply vinegar to the site.

SNAKEBITE – When I was quite young, a copperhead bit the mother of one of my high school classmates. It was miles to town to a doctor, and it would be necessary to hitch a team to the wagon to drive her there. A man grabbed and killed a chicken, tore it apart, and slapped it over the bite on her arm. Soon the hot meat of the chicken began to draw the venom out. No doctor was seen.

It is said that the Native Americans used a tea of echinacea for snakebite. It is supposed to stimulate the immune system. A neighbor mentioned that she has heard that park officials still use raw onion for snakebites. Others suggest carrying a small-mouth bottle with lots of non-iodized salt mixed in turpentine. Hold the mouth of the bottle tight against the bite site, and allow it to draw out the poison, which usually looks green in color. Other remedies include:

- Apply to the bite a hunk of salt or wad of tobacco mixed with saliva or water.
- Apply poultices of onion mixed with kerosene, which were left on until they turned green. At that time, apply a fresh poultice while on the way to a doctor. In fact, rush to find a doctor.

In case of snakebites, it is very important to be able to identify the type of snake. In this area, we have copperheads and rattlesnakes. A rattlesnake nearly always has rattles on its tail, while a copperhead has a hole in its head between the mouth and the ear area. The hole distinguishes it from a house snake, which has very similar coloring.

SPIDER BITES - We have two spiders locally that are very dangerous: the brown recluse and the black widow. The recluse has a violin-shaped marking on its back while the black widow's markings are a red or orange hourglass on the abdomen.

Our one-time experience with spider bites was when a black widow spider bit my brother. Mother beat an egg white, put it in a small-mouth bottle and held the bottle against the bite to draw out the poison. Being young at the time, I recall hearing my brother cry out in pain, but the remedy must have been successful.

To discourage spiders, one can spread cedar chips or spray with rubbing alcohol around a room.

TICKS - We had a case of a neighbor girl who became totally paralyzed for no apparent reason. The paralysis started at her feet and moved up toward her head. After it had reached her neck, a tick was found embedded on her spine. Once it was removed, she fully recovered.

We did not know that ticks carry various diseases such as Lyme Disease or Rocky Mountain Spotted Fever. We tried to check for ticks after we were in the woods before they could attach to us.

If a tick became attached to an animal, we put a lighted match to the backside of the tick, letting the heat make them release their hold. Because pulling them out sometimes caused infection, we washed the affected area with soap and then applied some iodine, alcohol or peroxide.

REPRODUCTIVE HEALTH

People in the mountains ranged from very proper to very crude in reference to discussing pregnancy and how one got that way. The proper ones would say someone was "in the family way" rather than saying someone was pregnant. Others, usually men, would say that a woman was "stung by a trouser worm" or "suffered from peter poisoning" or other very colorful expression. Pregnant women often would not go out of their houses because of their "conditions." If a pregnant woman answered a door, she showed only her face, because she did not want anyone to see her.

Nice women did not talk about sex, and information on the topic was often incorrect. My mother gave me only one piece of advice regarding birth control before I married. She told me she thought there was a "safe" time in the middle of the monthly period. About three or four months after my wedding, I took a chance during that time. Nine months later my first child was born. That could help to explain why my mother had eight children.

Despite a reluctance to talk about topics related to sex, it did, of course, occur. I sensed that people did it, but they were not supposed to enjoy it. I remember that my mother had a book about sex that she hid under some linens in our house. When I discovered the book, I realized it was too good to keep secret. I took it to school and read it with Ray Benson and Jessica

Robertson. When my mother learned what I had done, I certainly got "what for."

BIRTH CONTROL - Mountain people practiced "planned parenthood" in many ways. They had a very picturesque description for coitus interruptus - "pulling the dash before the butter comes." (A dash was the wooden implement used to churn butter.)

Some of the very early Smoky Mountain natives had a male birth control method that beat having a pill. An incision about one-inch long was cut into the urethra, near its junction with the scrotum. The edges of the wound were burned with a stone, and the wound was subsequently kept open by the introduction of a small piece of wood. When the wound healed, a permanent opening remained. During intercourse, the seminal discharge flew backward through this opening.

Some women ingested a few drops of turpentine to abort a pregnancy. A large amount of castor oil had to be taken along with the turpentine, because it caused great constipation. I never knew the dosage used for the abortions. I only knew one person personally who had missed a period and used the turpentine, but you hardly ask technical questions during such a conversation.

Some apparently also used slippery elm powder or pennyroyal to abort, but I never learned how those were used.

96

"FEMALE" PROBLEMS – There is some disagreement today as to the real symptoms associated with what women referred to as "the vapors." Because women did not discuss it further, no one was sure what symptoms they were experiencing. It could have been flatulence, but the term likely referred to PMS or symptoms of menopause. It may also have referred to feeling faint.

When I was a child, my mother used the wild roots, which grew nearby for whatever female problems ailed her. I remember going into the woods to dig black cohosh roots to make a tea for her to drink. Today we can buy black cohosh capsules in a bottle. Recommended dosage is one capsule up to three times daily. Or, 10 to 30 drops of extract daily in water. Black cohosh is said to induce menstrual periods, relieve cramps, facilitate labor and delivery, and relieve menopausal symptoms. I recently heard that excessive use of black cohosh might cause liver problems or other symptoms of poisoning, however.

Hot flash remedies include:

- Take one tablespoon apple cider vinegar and one tablespoon honey in six ounces of water at least three times daily.

- Drink chamomile, dill, sage, or catnip tea. The dosage is ½ teaspoon in warm water.

- Eat a cucumber daily.

- Massage the area between the thumb and index finger in a circular motion for five minutes.

MENSTRAUL PROBLEMS - A tea of evening primrose was supposed to reduce premenstrual symptoms. Some used peppermint or catnip tea to relieve cramps. Witch Hazel was used to treat excessive bleeding. We took the limbs of the witch hazel tree, cut them up, and made a tea to drink.

MORNING SICKNESS – Eating one or more pawpaws was said to reduce the nausea associated with morning sickness during pregnancy.

IMPOTENCE - Before pharmaceutical companies introduced the term erectile dysfunction (ED), we called it impotence, or we said someone lost his "nature." Ginseng was often used for this condition. The dosage was one-fourth teaspoon of powdered ginseng twice a month. Other remedies included:

- eating one-half cup of unprocessed shelled pumpkin or sunflower seeds daily;
- taking a bee pollen pill daily; or
- massaging the area in back of the ankle, about one and one-half inches above the shoe line of each foot to relax tension and stimulate circulation.

MASTURBATION – In my early years, we called this "self-abuse." Nice people certainly did not engage in the practice. At least they did not admit to it. I remember one time my mother showed me some pictures in a book showing what happened when one practiced masturbation. The book contained pictures of

98

children with very severe deformities. The implication was that this was what we would look like if we engaged in the activity.

We heard that if you did it, you would go blind. I understood there were some who thought they would try it until maybe they needed glasses.

YEAST INFECTION – Our remedies for vaginal yeast infections included douching with apple cider vinegar or bathing in a bath to which half a cup of salt and vinegar were added. I understand one doctor advised a patient to go naked for eight hours to cure her infection. My own doctor once told me to pull my drawers off and go to the mountains. I was a little skeptical.

RESPIRATORY AILMENTS

One old mountaineer asked to borrow some Copenhagen tobacco. He sniffed it deep on each side of his nose several times, and then started sneezing. After he sneezed some 15 times, he said his sinuses, which had been totally blocked, were clear.

My son says he knows of an old doctor, who used a very unusual method to clear sinuses. The doctor was said to have doubled up his fist and hit the patient right between the eyes as hard as he could. The sinus congestion cleared up as soon as the patient got over being mad. If this really happened, I wonder if the patient every returned.

ALLERGIES – We never used the word *allergies*, and we knew nothing about them. Every time we took our son Don to his grandparents' home in Wears Valley, he had an asthma attack. When he returned after helping his grandmother milk the cows, he was unable to breathe, but we did not see the connection.

What few mountain doctors we had always carried honeycomb in their little black medical bags. They gave it to sinus sufferers to chew like gum. The patient chewed it for 20 minutes every hour for 5-6 hours and then discarded it. This was continued for two days and then once each day for seven more days. To prevent sinus attacks or hay fever, some said to take two teaspoons of our local honey every day for 30 days before pollen season began.

ASTHMA - *Phthisic* was an old term used for asthma and other respiratory ailments. If you wish to try a good old hillbilly remedy, sworn to help asthma, do a one-minute dip of your entire body in our cold river water. It seems that this would make it worse, but I am just reporting what I heard.

Mountain folk cut a sourwood tree branch of a length equal to the height of an asthmatic child and stored this branch in the attic. When the child's height exceeded the length of the stick, his asthma was supposed to be cured.

Another treatment was to stand the child beside a fruit-bearing tree and measure his height. Boring a hole into the tree at that height, they placed a lock of the child's hair in the hole, and then plugged it. The child was supposed to have only one more bad attack.

Two members of my family actually received this second treatment. My sister Lillie Watson's hair was put into a chestnut tree. Grandmother Ida Myers followed this procedure with our son Don. She cut his hair and placed it in a cherry tree. Following this outlandish treatment, he had only one more bad asthma attack. I have often wondered if their "cure" was simply the power of suggestion. Maybe the child naturally outgrew asthma attacks. Other remedies include:

· Each day, chew honeycomb or take one teaspoon corn oil.

- Eat a raw potato or drink buttermilk daily.

- To soothe asthma coughs, drink a tea of evening primrose.

- Put the leaves of powdered ginseng, mullein, or rabbit tobacco in a pan. Place a hot coal on top of the leaves and inhale the smoke. Or, put the leaves in the sink, run hot water over them, and inhale the fumes.

- Keep a Chihuahua dog in the house to prevent attacks.

BRONCHITIS – Remedies I found for bronchitis include the following:

- Drink lots of water.

- Eat spicy foods such as garlic, onion, horseradish, or hot peppers.

- Drink a tea made of ½ -1 teaspoon of dried catnip in warm water.

- Stop all dairy products.

- Avoid sugar.

CHEST CONGESTION – One remedy for chest congestion was to put goose grease on a heated flannel cloth and hold on the chest. Onion poultices and mustard plasters were also used for chest ailments such as bad colds and coughs. The directions for making a mustard plaster are found in the section on childhood ailments. To make onion plasters, onions were baked and mashed into a clean cloth. They were then placed on the bare chest while still hot. This was supposed to bring blood to the surface of the skin.

Another remedy for chest congestion was to soak an eight-inch square of a brown paper bag in hot water and sprinkle with black pepper. Put the bag on the chest with the pepper next to the skin. When I have chest congestion, I put rice in a sock and tie the end of the sock. After heating it in the microwave, I place it on my chest instead of using a heating pad or hot water bottle.

COLDS and FLU – When we caught a cold or flu, we said we were "under the weather," "feeling poorly," or "ailin'." In about 1919, my mother and dad avoided the devastating flu epidemic. They said they stayed in bed with jars of hot water and sweated for 2-4 hours. This would be like using hot water bottles or sitting in a sauna today. Afterwards, they were very careful not to become chilled. I have heard that raising the body temperature to 102° increases white blood cells and makes them more active against infections.

Garlic, zinc, and echinacea were used for cold and flu treatment. When someone was suffering from a cold, Granny Myers put an onion in ashes in the fireplace and roasted it. Not only did it taste good, it was supposed to ease the symptoms. Some people put sulfur in the center of an onion before burying it in the ashes.

We can thank our Native Americans for introducing us to a new-world herb, boneset. For flu, which they called "break bone fever" or "bone breaking fever," boneset relieved congestion, coughing, and loosened phlegm. Boneset can cause liver damage if too much is ingested. It also can have side effects, which include muscular tremors, weakness, and severe constipation.

A cure I collected many years ago came from a very old newspaper article. It said that an ear-nose-and-throat specialist had cured most of his patients' colds by an amazingly simple therapy. He had patients immerse their forearms in a basin of hot water 104-113° F for 30-60 minutes. He said soaking the forearms increased blood circulation and temperatures in the walls of nasal passages, which, in turn, wards off new cold-causing germs. He claimed a cure rate of 75% for his grandmother's remedy, which for centuries had been used in some of Europe's rural areas.

Another cold remedy was elderberry. In ancient times, elderberry trees were believed to bring good luck or protect against evil spirits and disease. For that reason, they were often planted near houses. Parts of the tree, other than flowers and berries, are considered poisonous, and the berries should always be cooked. The flowers are believed to be good for colds and flu. Pennyroyal, another plant, which can be dangerous, was also used for colds and flu.

One woman with whom I spoke said she snuffed - or sniffed - up salt water into her sinuses and declared she has not had a cold in the past ten years. I recently heard a medical report on the radio saying that saline solution sprayed into nostrils actually helps to prevent colds and relieve cold symptoms.

While I was visiting with David Ethridge, I asked him about his most memorable medical remedy when he was a child. He immediately touched both forefingers and thumbs together, making a circle about six inches in diameter. He said his family used a tin can about that size and put boiling water and then a little turpentine in it. Placing a newspaper or towel over the head, they breathed the fumes to stop a cold or flu dead in its tracks.

A woman overhearing our conversation added that when one of her family had a chest cold or flu symptoms, they painted colored iodine on the chest and back, and it cured them. She said they made their nose drops out of beet juice (three parts juice to 1 part honey.) She said she has never seen a doctor for any medications. They always made their own. Other remedies for colds and flu are listed below.

- Many early settlers ingested pine resin to help them breathe better. Others gathered short twigs and needles from pine trees, put them in an enamel pan, and simmered three or four hours. After straining out the solid pieces, they mixed the liquid with lots of honey and took one teaspoon per day. It is said the Native Americans introduced this remedy.

- To relieve chills and cold symptoms, eat chili peppers or drink a tea made of dried peppers.

- Eat chicken soup or drink peppermint tea.

- Sniff horseradish or inhale the vapors of ammonia or vinegar.

This one sounds very unusual, but I collected it, too. Some have said that tying a red ribbon or scarf around the left wrist and neck, or wearing nothing but white for three days will help a cold. I have my doubts about that one.

A slice of garlic put in each window in the house is supposed to keep away cold germs.

COUGHS - No cough syrup in drug stores today compares with the wonderful old red clover tea my mother made after I had coughed for several weeks. It tasted so good, and it stopped my coughing immediately! Some used the pine resin remedy described in the previous section for coughs. Other remedies are:

- Sip a mixture of one teaspoon ginger and a bit of sugar mixed in one cup of hot water.

- Eat cooked red cabbage mixed with honey.

- Cut the bark from a wild cherry tree. After washing the bark, put it in an enamel or stainless steel pot to boil for 30 minutes. Strain, add sugar, and boil to syrup. Take one teaspoon about every four hours.

- Put a whole onion in milk and boil it for 10-15 minutes so that the juice of the onion will seep out in the milk. Take out the onion, and drink the milk.

- Black cohosh, the herb used for many female problems, is also used to treat long-term coughs when drunk in a tea.

- After taking three rounds of antibiotics from the doctor for a bad cough recently, I tried the very old mountain remedy of "rock and rye," rock candy in rye whiskey. It cured me.

EARACHE - For earache, our family used what we called sweet oil, which always helped. We warmed the oil just a bit and poured it into the ears. I was recently getting ready to pay a high price for sweet oil when the pharmacist whispered to me to put it back on the shelf. He said to go to the grocery and buy some olive oil. Before returning the bottle to the pharmacy shelf, I noted that it read "100% olive oil." Having the name *sweet oil* costs a lot more. In addition to using sweet oil, we heated rice tied in a sock and applied heat to the ears. We also blew smoke into the ears to relieve the pain.

Allie Newman Maples, wife of the late Bruce Maples of Gatlinburg, relayed perhaps the most unusual treatment for earache I have heard. She told of crying for several days with earache when she was a child. After keeping her parents awake several nights, they decided the situation was critical enough to take her to Sevierville to see a doctor. En route to Sevierville, they met the doctor. Because he had nothing in his little black bag to treat earache, he told them what to do. He said to catch some of her urine, and put a few drops in her ears. The situation was so bad by then that she agreed to it. Believe it or not, she said

108

the pain stopped, and she never had another earache. I was a little skeptical about this story, but I recently read that others reported this as an accepted mountain remedy.

HOARSENESS – For hoarseness or loss of voice, we usually gargled with warm salted water. A house cleaner, who once worked at our house, taught me to make black pepper tea - black pepper in hot water. We also used white rock candy dissolved in water. Other remedies include:

- Add the juice of one lemon and a small amount of sugar to the white of one beaten egg. Take a teaspoon of the mixture every half-hour.
- Drink a mixture of approximately one tablespoon of honey and 1/4 cup apple cider vinegar.
- Sniff horseradish or eat some on a cracker.

PNEUMONIA – When I had pneumonia as a child, a doctor told my mother there was nothing more he could do for me. She immediately made a hot poultice using cornmeal with lots of onions and put it on my chest as hot as I could stand it. As soon as it cooled, she made another poultice and applied it. This continued for several hours. I survived.

Other people warmed a mixture of turpentine, grease, and Vick's salve and applied it to the chest. Then they covered it with a warm woolen cloth and repeated the treatment as needed to keep the mixture warm.

Another remedy for pneumonia used corn whiskey diluted with water, to which black pepper and sugar were added. The dose was one teaspoon for a child and ¼ cup for an adult every hour.

SINUS PROBLEMS – I recall the incident of a child who had not been able to breathe through his nose for four months. He was given honeycomb to chew. After four or five minutes he said, "I can breathe through my nose."

Doctors in the mountains also used tincture of merthiolate on a swab pushed deep into both sinus cavities. However, they cautioned not to use this more than once per month.

Among the foods we believed to be helpful for sinus problems were raw spinach, fresh carrots, grape juice, garlic, onions, fresh mint, and radishes. Inhaling the smoke from coffee grounds in a pipe was also a favorite remedy.

I have put two tablespoons or more of brandy in a cup of boiling water. Then, I surround the cup with my hands, alternately breathing the steam through my mouth and nose. I continue for 15 minutes. Afterwards, one can just drink the brandy and feel fine.

For sinus headache, put cold compresses on the forehead, and soak the feet in hot water. This is supposed to draw blood to the lower extremities and relieve a headache.

SORE THROAT – To ease sore throat discomfort, add 1/8 teaspoon black pepper or three tablespoons apple cider vinegar to one cup of hot water and sip the mixture. Other remedies are:

- At bedtime, take a teaspoon of honey, and let it trickle down the throat. Do not drink any liquid following this as the honey helps to kill germs.

- Drink warm sage tea.

- Dissolve one-third teaspoon baking soda in water and sip repeatedly all day.

- Gargle with Coca-Cola.

- A favorite gargle for sore throat was a mixture of one teaspoon salt, one teaspoon soda, and a few drops of iodine. This remedy, called SSI, was one of our favorites when I worked at the hospital.

- I prefer gargling with 100% hydrogen peroxide. Afterwards, I rinse it out well.

TONSILLITIS - Old timers called it *quinsy*. A flaxseed (linseed) poultice, made like a mustard poultice, was applied to the throat for tonsillitis. Another remedy was to paint the outside of the throat with iodine. The popular herb, echinacea has also been used to treat tonsillitis. Another suggested remedy is propolis.

TUBERCULOSIS – Tuberculosis or TB was once common in this area. It was often called consumption or tubercular consumption. Checking Dr. Pierce's book, he offered a mail-

111

order remedy called Dr. Pierce's Golden Medical Discovery. He indicated that at the time his book was written (1895), one in every 323 people died annually of consumption. He said perhaps as much as 1/7 of the deaths each year were from consumption.

My dad's first wife, Sophia (called Sophie), died with TB. I do not know what treatment she would have received. Back then, they knew to put the patient out in the sun and to apply mustard poultices. I understand taking doses of cod liver oil or eating watercress were also used to treat consumption.

Another remedy was mullein tea. Dried mullein leaves were steeped in water. Using this tea for three to six months was said to cure TB. Another remedy was to pour boiling hot water and any flavor of brandy into a cup. Holding your hands around the cup, breathe the steam for a few minutes. I understand that when Edgar Cayce's wife was dying of TB, he had her breathe the fumes of hot water mixed with brandy and she recovered.

SKIN PROBLEMS

I remember skin diseases being quite common in my childhood. There was baker's itch, barber's itch, washerwoman's itch, bricklayer's itch, grocer's itch, fever blisters, cold sores, shingles, brow-shingles, milk-crust, tetter, etc. When I was a child, I had tetter, which referred to a variety of skins problems having itching and eruptions. To cure it, we went to the woods, dug some bloodroot, and made a tea. After this was applied to the skin, the tetter was cured with one application. Coal tar soap was often used in those days. It was also used as a shampoo and to treat and kill head lice. I understand it is fairly expensive now if you can find it. However, I recently read that soaps with a high concentration of coal tar can be carcinogenic.

I once read that a football coach in North Carolina just across the mountain said the following words over injured team members.

> "Bruise, thou shall not heat,
> Bruise, thou shall not sweat,
> Bruise thou shall not run,
> No more than the Virgin Mary
> shall bring forth another son,
> (while doing the sign of the cross)
> In the name of God the Father,
> In the name of God the son,
> In the name of God, The Holy Ghost! Amen.

At first, the boys made great sport of this ceremony and called the coach a "crackpot." After some of them experienced beneficial results, it is said they later came to him and requested it.

ATHLETE'S FOOT – As children, we tied a wool or cotton string around our toes if we got an infection or little white blisters between and around them. Others called the blisters "cow itch"; we called it athlete's foot. It may not have been athletes' foot, but our remedy for it certainly worked. Donna Myers, my daughter-in-law, could not believe it when my son Don told her about this remedy, so he called me and put Donna on the phone for me to verify his story.

I have also heard that soaking feet in vinegar or spraying vinegar on the toes works to cure the little white blisters. A third remedy is to mix baking soda with water to make a paste and rub that between the toes.

BOILS - OR CARBUNCLES - When a boil had two heads, it was called a carbuncle. When boils started, we applied turpentine to them, which prevented them from developing any further. Hot poultices of flaxseeds were also applied, especially after something was lanced.

Other remedies designed to draw pus out of a boil are bacon fat or small amounts of scraped raw potato bound on the boil. My choice is a paste made of slippery elm bark. Others suggest using echinacea.

A patent medicine we used for many skin problems is a black salve known as Ichthammol. This product is so old-fashioned that a pharmacist must special order it today. It costs less than two dollars and has great drawing power. Our family has used it for more than 50 years.

BRUISES – We did not use the chant used by the football coach for bruises, but we had many other remedies. One remedy we did use was to alternately apply two wash clothes - one dipped in very hot water and the other dipped in very cold water. We wrung out the very hot cloth and put it on the bruise for three minutes. We applied the very cold cloth for one minute. This process was repeated at least four times. The hot water brings blood to the area while the cold takes it away.

One of the most common remedies for bruises was to apply to the skin a couple of times a day the juice from black walnut hulls or a liquid made from boiling black walnut leaves or bark. The plant was also useful for eczema, herpes, psoriasis, warts, skin parasites, and shingles.

Other remedies to reduce bruising include applying grated onion mixed with salt or the inside of a pawpaw peel.

Eating citrus fruit is supposed to help with bruise prevention.

BURNS - Hill folk "blew the fire out of burns." In this mountain ceremony, a burn doctor started by passing his or her hands slowly, with palms down and open, three times over the burn. Blowing their breathe gently, they followed the hands as they passed over the burned area. Placing their heads over the burn, they turned so the breath followed the hands away from the victim's body and away from the healer. They continued this treatment silently for up to 30 minutes. Sometimes during the treatment they repeated, "There came an angel from the east. Bring frost and fire. In frost, out fire. In the name of the Father, the Son, and the Holy Ghost." Healers were known to work for two weeks on a badly burned person. They would put only talcum powder or baby powder on a severe burn. They did not bind it with any dressing or let water touch the burn.

One day, while stirring apple butter, two big blobs popped out on my hand. Just to see if one could blow the fire out of a burn, I quickly washed off the apple butter and decided to blow the worst and bigger spot while leaving the other one alone. (I did not use any ceremony.) For perhaps thirty minutes, I continued to blow my breath on the larger spot.

Today, I have a scar where the lesser burn was located, while there is no scar where I blew on the larger spot. Perhaps the oxygen or the cooling helped.

I have found slippery elm powder to be a very good treatment for burns. When our second son Glenn was ten months old, he fell while standing in his highchair. His hand went into a boiling hot bowl of gravy I had just set on the table. Washing his hand quickly in cold water, I applied a very thick coating of slippery elm powder mixed with Vaseline. I left the salve on overnight. The next day, I could find no sign of this terrible burn.

Other remedies for mild burns, including sunburn, are apple cider vinegar, aloe, yogurt, damp baking soda, iced milk mixed with salt, the juice of a slice of cucumber, the liquid from boiled chestnut leaves, or the juice of fresh ginger. Some extract the juice of a whole leek plant and use it as a salve for burns.

Thick layers of soap were spread over acid burns. Salt water was used for rope burns. A remedy for a burned tongue was to apply granulated sugar or vanilla.

A doctor told me that honey applied to burns is the best remedy there is. He said that every family should keep a quart of honey in the house for use in case of burns. Others have used propolis, which comes from beehives for burns.

CHAPPED HAND - A mixture of equal parts of glycerin and bay rum, which is distilled from bayberry leaves, was used for chapped hands. Rose oil was added to give it a pleasant scent. All-vegetable shortening is considered an excellent skin moisturizer, and it is much cheaper than most brand-name moisturizers.

We purchased Cloverine salve for chapped hands. It looked good enough to eat, but it was known for its ability to cure chapped hands. It was one of my favorites due to its pleasant smell.

COLD FEET - Our Cherokee neighbors taught us to put red pepper in our socks for cold feet. Rather than wearing warm socks all the time, one can stand in the bathtub, turn on hot water for one minute and then cold water for one minute. This is supposed to help regulate temperatures in the feet.

CORNS AND CALLUSES – Many remedies were suggested for corns and calluses.

- Castor oil, lard, sweet oil, or vinegar can be applied to soften corns and calluses.

- Some people squeezed juice from dandelion stems and continued to apply the juice until the corns were gone.

- Apply white vinegar in a poultice several nights.

- Tape a slice of raw onion on corns or calluses every night for three or four weeks until they disappear.

118

· Today, I have heard to use WD-40. I do not know how it is used.

FEET – For thirty minutes or more, bathe uncomfortable or burning feet and legs in fresh crushed tomatoes mixed with water.

FEVER BLISTERS OR COLD SORES – Drink a tea made of yellowroot or pieces of a witch hazel limb. A more exotic remedy was to put your own earwax on cold sores. Today, some suggest painting them with colorless nail polish.

DOG DAYS – Everyone is familiar with the term "dog days," the hottest and muggiest part of the summer. We believed that wounds or sores would not heal easily during that time. We applied blackberry leaves or peach leaves mixed with lard to heal sores that otherwise did not heal during dog days.

While working at the Gatlinburg Medical Center one summer, many of our patients were having serious problems with infections that would not heal. The doctor was being very critical of our nurses and was blaming them for being careless.

After I listened to the doctor rant for a while, I interrupted him saying, "Doc, don't you know that it's dog days?" Probably exasperated, he turned and left the room without another word.

ECZEMA - Folklore told us that carrying a potato in our pockets cured eczema. However, I would more likely go with the bloodroot we dug on the little hill back of the pasture field to cure it. The sap of the bloodroot plant is orange red (giving the plant its name.) Black walnut juice is also recommended for many skin irritations including eczema, psoriasis, warts, and shingles. Other suggested herbal remedies are echinacea or burdock.

FELONS - are not criminals. They are abscesses on fingers or toes, usually around the nail. My mother had many felons on her fingers, perhaps due to using excessively hot dish and wash water. She cut a hole in the end of a lemon large enough to insert her finger. Then, she wore this lemon on her finger two to three days or until the infection was gone.

FROSTBITE - When my mother was a child, she attended a one-room school located in the Sugarlands, south of Gatlinburg. Before potbelly stoves, they often left a hole in the center of a room, where an open fire was built. Sitting around this fire, my mother developed frostbite on her heels. Her parents soaked her frostbitten heels in hot water to which they added chestnut leaves. Then they cut out the heels of her shoes so she could return to school.

A rather unusual remedy is to soak a hornet's nest in water and bathe the affected area with the water. Other remedies included applying witch hazel, sweet oil, propolis, or aloe to the injury.

Or, they mixed turpentine and salt into a salve and applied twice daily for several days.

HIVES – An interesting treatment was to wrap a person suffering from hives in a solid red blanket. It seems strange, but with information about different colors retaining or reflecting light and heat, I like to believe there is something to it. I have seen the difference in ripening when tomatoes are wrapped in different colors of clothe.

INGROWN TOENAIL - For infection and soreness of ingrown toenails, cut a big hole in a raw onion and put the toe into the onion. Bind it on to the toe overnight. Other remedies include soaking in Epsom salts mixed in warm water, or mixing honey and propolis and binding on the toes.

Stuff some cotton under the nail to lift it up and let it grow out. To prevent ingrown toenails, cut straight across when trimming the nails.

ITCHING - When one itched without eruptions, it was relieved by applying vinegar or a mixture of whiskey and salt to the itching skin. They would also let a slug crawl across the itching spot. That remedy, I did not try.

ITCH (SCABIES) - This highly contagious bug can be transferred by handling any item an affected person has touched.

121

Since scabies was so highly contagious, it was not considered a disgrace to get it, just a disgrace to keep it.

I must confess I was a victim when I was very young. Mother greased me from head to foot with sulfur mixed with lard. Then she made me stand in my altogether, or, as some would say, "nekked," in front of a hot fire that baked in the sulfur. I do not recall if this treatment was repeated. I remember that we had to burn all clothing and bedding that came in contact with the sulfur, as that odor cannot be removed. We also used pokeroot or dog hobble to kill the itch. It was smeared head to toe and worn for three days.

In addition to suggesting his mail order treatment of Dr. Pierce's Pleasant Pellets for itch, Dr. Pierce said to add *"half an ounce of blood-root to half a pint of vinegar, steep moderately for two hours, strain and paint the affected parts once or twice daily with the liquid. A tea of black walnut leaves, applied as a lotion to the affected parts, has also proved beneficial."*

PSORIASIS – Epsom salts was used to treat psoriasis. It was mixed with water and applied as a paste, or it was added to a bath. When soaking in a tub with Epsom salts, it is important not to allow the water temperature to fall below 98° F., as body heat pulls poison back into the pores of the skin.

Another remedy is a mixture of two tablespoons of flaxseed oil and one half cup of cottage cheese eaten once daily until psoriasis clears. A third remedy is the juice of black walnut hulls rubbed on the skin twice daily. Burdock has also been suggested.

RASH - I remember that Mother told my sister Ollie that her husband should use alcohol for his galded (rash) condition among his privates. That just happened to be the wrong application for a raw condition. You should have heard the description of Wilson's race to the branch (creek) some 500 yards behind the house. He tried to run with his pants down around his feet so that he could sit in the cold mountain water. I would expect that Mother avoided that son-in-law for quite some time after that error.

Less extreme remedies called for bathing in a warm bath with baking soda, apple cider vinegar, or oatmeal (tied in a sock or panty hose) added to the water.

SHINGLES - A friend said she lay in the floor and screamed with pain from shingles. Her condition lasted for weeks. She learned that, to avoid this horrible suffering, one should get to a doctor immediately when confronted with shingles. Home remedies I have collected include:

· Place the bark or leaves of the black walnut in boiling water and allow to simmer. Apply the liquid to the affected area.

Or one can apply the juice of the hulls twice daily to relieve the pain.

- Grind oatmeal into a fine powder, or tie it into a very thin cloth such as cheesecloth or panty hose, and add to a warm bath. Soak in bath water for about 30 minutes. This can be hung from the spigot to allow the oatmeal to disperse in the water.

- Another remedy to relieve itching suggests bathing for about 20 minutes in a warm bath to which a hand full of cornstarch has been added.

- Various single products have been suggested for shingles. They include applying witch hazel, geranium oil, Phillips Milk of Magnesia, pepper sauce such as Tabasco, or the liquid from the aloe plant to the affected area.

- Apply a paste of baking soda or Epsom salts mixed with water.

- Crush two Bayer aspirin tablets into a powder and mix with Cutex nail polish remover. Apply the mixture to the affected area with a cotton ball and let dry for several hours. Do not use if allergic to aspirin.

- Apply a thin coat of Colgate Toothpaste over dried pepper sauce such as Tabasco. The glycerin in toothpaste is said to reduce the burning discomfort; the pepper is supposed to act as an analgesic.

- Fill a Ziploc bag with ice cubes, wrap in a towel, and rub the affected areas.

SUNBURN - (See burns.) As with minor burns of other types, apply apple cider vinegar or baking soda dissolved in water. Tie oatmeal into an old sock, and place the sock in a cool bath. For sun poisoning, apply vinegar and soda, or wash with Palmolive soap and then apply pure Vaseline to the skin.

We did not know that it was necessary to protect our skin from anything other than the discomfort of sunburn. We simply wore long sleeves and big hats. We were told that sweet oil and vinegar mixed half-and-half could prevent sunburn. When my son lived in Myrtle Beach, he was told that taking aspirin before going in the sun would prevent sunburn. I seemed to help.

WARTS - Charming warts was a great pastime in the mountains. Children with warts would seek out a wart charmer at church gatherings, family reunions, and other events. Adults occasionally had their warts charmed as well. Charmers, usually older people, who kept the process secret, would pass the secret only to members of the opposite sex. I could not bear to be left out, so I found a man willing to tell me how this was done.

The charmer used his or her finger to draw circles around the wart, first seven times in a clockwise direction and then seven times in a counterclockwise direction. As the charmer went around the wart with the finger, he or she moved his lips and counted. If the wart did not come off in two or three weeks, the "patient" was to return for a second treatment.

My son-in-law, Ed Boyer, tells that when he was young, his grandfather, Andrew Dunn, took him to visit a man, who said he would remove some warts on his hand. The man found a small bunch of pine needles and measured the width of the warts with them. Then, he cut the pine needles this length and buried them in a glass jar. He told Ed to forget about them; they would go away. They did.

We had many more remedies for removing warts, which I have listed below.

- Old-timers used a single application of linseed (flaxseed) oil and Podophyllum in lanolin. They kept this on for seven days to remove warts.

- Apply castor oil or a mixture of baking soda and castor oil for nine nights. Rub the inside of a pawpaw peel on the wart each day for a few days.

- Steal your mother's dishrag and bury it. When the rag rots, the warts will be gone. Put a slice of potato on a wart; then bury the potato.

- Rub the wart with a sliced onion. Bury the onion. When the onion rots, the warts are supposed to be gone.

- I was told to cut my wart until it bled, rub the wart with an ear of corn, and then feed the corn to the chickens. I followed this advice, and my wart eventually disappeared. Some say if you do nothing, the wart will still disappear.

- Recently, I read that you can cover a wart with Elmer's Glue. When the glue is dry, peel it off the skin. Repeat two or three times per day.

- Here I sit with duct tape on some warts.

VETERINARY CONCERNS

William Flannigan, a neighbor, mentioned the serious threat of mad dogs (hydrophobia) during our early childhood. When I was a child, I remember my mother and dad discussing a man in Gatlinburg who contracted rabies. He was chained outside near where the Charles Ogle store was located. Discussion of that poor man, chained outside, and then dying like that sure sounded horrible to me. The place he was tied is now the 50-store Mountain Mall at the forks of the road where the river road branches off the main street.

I only saw one mad dog, as we called them. Our dear old Limber had been missing some two or three weeks when we saw him coming home foaming at the mouth and his tail tucked between his legs. I am not sure if that description told me he was suffering from hydrophobia or if it was that Mother so quickly closed the back gate to our yard. Either way, Mother grabbed her old shotgun and shot our beloved dog. She was never known to miss the target. Seeing our dog come home to die and mother having to end his suffering was a very traumatic experience for me.

If a dog believed to have rabies bit someone, a red-hot poker or live coals were applied to the site. Sometimes a knife was used to cut away the raw surface of a bite. Alcohol, ammonia or iodine was applied, if available.

CATS – Pennyroyal is supposed to prevent fleas on cats and other animals. We never used it, however. Putting a teaspoon of corn oil on a cat's food once a week is supposed prevent hairballs.

CHICKENS – A neighbor told me how his mother doctored their sick chickens. She soaked a feather in kerosene. Then, holding a chicken's bill open, she rammed the kerosene-soaked feather down its throat and pulled it back out. The neighbor said the chickens soon got well.

Sassafras poles make good chicken roosts. The poles were supposed to prevent chicken mites.

COWS - Our most rambunctious milk cow, Daisy, choked on apples almost every summer. To save Daisy's life, we kept a broom handle with a rag tied on the end to push those apples on down her throat. She never learned, so we were always prepared for another episode. Jerze, the other milk cow, ate the same apples but never had any such problems.

When one of our cows ceased to chew her cud, it was called both "holler" horn or "holler" tail (hollow). A number of remedies were used. Dad held turpentine to their navels as a remedy. Others wrapped the horn in a flannel cloth soaked in turpentine for a few days. Some split the tail and inserted mixtures of things like salt, pepper, soot and/or turpentine. Some bored holes in the horn and poured salt water in the hole.

Another remedy was to pour hot Watkins liniment down the cow's throat. Watkins Liniment, which contained camphor, was first sold in the 1800s and was used by many farmers. The hot liniment contained hot pepper, which relieved pain. It is still sold today, I understand.

We always fed our cows flaxseeds, which we called linseeds, along with their regular feed. I am not sure why. When cows are pregnant, add at least two ounces of apple cider vinegar to their feed each day to keep them healthy. If calves chew on wood, mix one ounce of apple cider vinegar to one gallon of water for them to drink.

DOGS - We were never allowed to feed our dogs biscuits, because they were said to cause dogs to have "fits." When I was younger, we cured mange on our dogs by applying burnt cylinder oil to the affected area. I have also heard that spraying a dog with WD-40 cures mange.

We removed ticks from a dog by lighting a match or candle and holding it to the back end of a tick until it released its hold and could be pulled off the dog.

LAMENESS - Mix one-tablespoon turpentine, one egg yolk, and one-tablespoon apple cider vinegar. Rub in well. This remedy is useful for animals and people. Various liniments, such as Watkins liniment, were also used to treat lameness.

SKUNK ODOR – Occasionally our dogs came home after a losing encounter with a skunk. While we usually just tried to avoid the animal until the smell went away naturally, I have since learned that you can use tomato juice or mix a cup of soda in hydrogen peroxide to shampoo the dog.

WOUNDS – Old timers used kerosene to speed healing for just about any kind of wound on themselves and their animals.

VISION AND HEARING

I recall my grandfather Ephraim Ogle had a hearing problem such that we had to at him. Back then, old folks had a hollow tapered bugle or horn that one talked into. I do not know where his ear horn came from unless it was from a dehorned cow. Otherwise, it would have been purchased, which I doubt. It was large at one end and very small at the other. Some hearing aid!!! But it helped.

As people aged, little really helped with loss of vision or hearing. Cataract surgery was unheard of. There were no hearing aids. Glasses were not commonly worn. I have listed below some of the conditions and treatments associated with vision and hearing.

BLACK EYES - Most remedies for black eyes involve putting something cool on the eye. One treatment was simply to cut a potato in half and hold it on the eye. Others included applying grated cucumber, scrapped or grated red potato, bruised peach leaves, or a mixture of shortening and salt. I remember that for many years television would show someone with a piece of raw beef on their eye after a fight. This was apparently supposed to heal a black eye. We would not have used meat that way.

CATARACTS - Today, we know to avoid UV light rays. A hospital administrator told me about a woman sent home to wait for cataract surgery. When she returned, the cataracts were gone.

After much urging, she confessed that an old mountain woman told her to put brown sugar in her eyes. The hospital administrator added that the drops given after cataract surgery contained brown sugar in solution.

Doctors recommend that nothing of this type go into the eyes because of concerns for scratching the cornea and introducing infection. They also say that a topical substance such as this will not reach the lens of the eye. I have tried brown sugar, however, to keep my cataracts at bay. It really hurts for a couple of minutes, but I found it helpful to splash cold water on closed eyelids. In the last few years, I have seen three new cataract preventive solutions using brown sugar come on the market. Some think including apple cider vinegar in your diet helps to prevent cataracts.

EARS – We were told never to put anything larger than an elbow in our ears. I guess that was meant to prevent us from sticking anything in our ears. My aural rehabilitationist, my ear specialist, says mineral oil poured into the ear is best to bring out earwax.

EYES - For cinders or other debris in the eyes, chop an onion and let the tears wash it out. We also sometimes put a flaxseed in our eyes to gather up dust or other foreign bodies.

For granulated eyelids or inflamed eyes, apply a weak solution of boric acid, a poultice of scrapped potato, or castor oil packs.

132

Years ago, pharmacies sold glass eye cups to use with liquid eye solutions. With bottled eye drops, you do not see these any more.

HEARING LOSS - Until you lose the major part of your hearing, you have no idea the effect it has on your life. I paid a small fortune for digital hearing aids that are supposed to adjust by computer. Every sound echoes through my head. I cannot sing. My words come out with something I did not intend to say. Being in groups is devastating. I see everyone laugh, but I have no idea what was funny. The only time the hearing aids are helpful is when I am talking to just one person alone in a quiet room.

Treatments I have found to reverse hearing loss do not sound very promising, but here they are.

- Stand on tiptoes with arms stretched high above the head and force several yawns.
- Here I may sound a little crazy, but there are those out there who swear by this practice. They say that pinching your middle fingers on each hand for five minutes, four times per day will help restore hearing.

NIGHT BLINDNESS - Eat blueberries to restore night vision, or put a drop of raw honey in the eye. The honey hurts for a couple of minutes, but splashing cold water on them soothes the discomfort.

Some also consider bilberry tea or capsules useful in preventing night blindness reporting that World War II Royal Air Force pilots used it for nighttime missions. A recent study by the U.S. Navy found no effect, and it does not appear to be well known in the RAF itself. Some studies indicate bilberry can reverse the effects of conditions such as macular degeneration, however.

STY - In the early days, the only remedy for a sty was to use an eyewash made from parsley leaves, which were boiled in water and steeped for 10-15 minutes. This one you may not believe. Rub a sty three times with a gold wedding ring. Another supposed remedy I ran across recently is even more unbelievable: rub the tail of a black cat over the sty.

PINKEYE OR CONJUNCTIVITIS – Straining out the seeds, squeeze the juice of a freshly cut tomato into the eye. Do not use canned tomato juice. This remedy is said to be an absolute cure.

- Rub a drop of castor oil squeezed onto a sterile pad across affected eyelids.
- To clear up pinkeye in a couple of days, apply a poultice of grated raw red potato or grated apple to closed eyes.
- Put chamomile flowers in just-boiled water. Steep for five minutes. Strain through unbleached muslin. Then use the solution as an eye wash.

SUN BLINDNESS - Eat sunflower seeds every day for sun blindness. Since no one has ever seen a rabbit wearing glasses, be sure to eat your carrots.

GENERAL REMEDIES AND TREATMENTS

In my early years, it was poultices instead of pills and herbs instead of injections. Before the days of pharmacies, we used the ingredients we found around us. Over the generations, different remedies were found to work for different conditions.

In the fall, members of the family gathered and dried leaves of various plants such as catnip, boneset, chamomile, and sage. These dried leaves were placed in bags and stored for the winter.

When someone was under the weather, a friend or relative was always willing to suggest a treatment. They would often say to use "a right smart" or "just a tad." They might tell someone to take an amount that would fit on the head of a dime or nickel. We also used the more conventional measures of teaspoon and tablespoon when describing dosages.

We sometimes ate particular foods to cure or prevent diseases or conditions. Perhaps the most important "health" foods were bee pollen, garlic, flaxseed, nuts, ginger and ginseng.

Many substances were noted for their medicinal qualities. In this chapter, I will discuss those remedies that were most commonly used or were used for so many different conditions that we would consider them indispensable.

ASAFETIDA - Some in our area actually used the very old remedy, asafetida, also known as "Devil's Dung." I never saw it or smelled it, but early mountain folk wore it around their necks. Its presence was supposed to ward off illness. Perhaps just keeping others at a distance was its chief benefit. Our family enjoyed telling the story of the farmer who wore his asafetida bag when he made a trip to the store. Rain fell on him; then the sun came out. This apparently activated the odor of his asafetida.

When he arrived home, his children ran to meet him and to receive the candy he promised to bring them. The children were so repelled by the odor that they ran back to their mother, holding their noses. One of the children exclaimed, "Ma, Paw's dead and don't know it!"

ALFALFA – Because alfalfa is usually used as cattle fodder, it is not often considered for its medicinal properties. However, it has been used for arthritis, urinary tract infections, an appetite stimulant, and overall tonic. It has also been used as a laxative and diuretic.

APPLES – are supposed to be good for constipation and diarrhea. They have been used to regulate blood sugar, lower cholesterol, and they are a traditional remedy for rheumatism.

BAYBERRY BARK – (Wax Myrtle) was one of the most versatile plants available. It was drunk in a hot tea at the first sign of a cold, cough, or flu. It is believed to be a great mouthwash, soothing for sore gums, and good for circulation. Bayberry is supposed to reduce the swelling of varicose veins, and it is one of the oldest remedies for hemorrhoids. In case of poisoning, it has been used to induce vomiting.

BURDOCK – Burdock is supposed to be a blood purifier. It is considered a diuretic, because when consumed in a tea, it causes sweating. It has been used to treat arthritis, rheumatism, eczema, psoriasis, measles, and canker sores. The dosage was 10 to 25 drops in water. I do not know how often it was to be used. Burdock was said to help if a rabid dog bit someone. I would definitely not rely on it for rabies prevention or treatment today.

CHAMOMILE – or pineapple weed, has many uses. Drunk as a tea, it is supposed to be great for nervous stomach, insomnia, rheumatism, toothache, digestion and gas. Chamomile is generally recognized to calm the nerves. When the leaves are crushed and applied to the skin, chamomile relieves itching and helps to heal sores. Take one to three capsules daily or up to one teaspoon dried chamomile in ½-cup warm water. In addition to its medicinal properties, it can be used as a mouthwash and to highlight blonde hair.

ECHINACEA - EK-in-nasia was used by the Cherokees as a snakebite remedy and as a general cure-all for infections. The first Echinacea was brewed as a tea. Only in recent years has it been available in capsules. Folks began to use it to reduce the effects of colds in the 1930's. Some research groups have claimed their testing of echinacea proved it to be worthless, but I can say it has always helped me when I started to get a cold. Echinacea proponents suggest varying research results occur because of differences in the quality of ingredients studied.

Echinacea is listed as one of the twelve most powerful herbs, and it has been studied perhaps more than any herbal remedy in the world. It has been used it to treat fevers, cholera, boils, abscesses, ulcers, poison ivy and oak, acne, headaches, tonsillitis, respiratory infections, bronchitis, measles, chicken pox, scarlet fever, eczema, appendicitis, snakebites, venereal diseases, and others. Echinacea should never be taken during pregnancy.

EPSOM SALTS – Epsom salts have been used since about the 1600's when a farmer in England noticed that the water on his farm seemed to heal scratches and sores on his cattle. We have used Epsom salts as a laxative, for relaxing muscles, and relieving sprains. When my daughter began premature labor, she was surprised to learn that the intravenous medication they gave her was magnesium sulfate - Epsom salts. I have bathed my legs in Epsom salts in very warm water when I have discomfort that seemed to be associated with blood clots. When used in a bath, it is important to remember that Epsom salts are absorbed into the skin. Therefore, the water should never be allowed to become cooler than body temperature.

EVENING PRIMROSE - was an old remedy for "cradle cap" (eczema.) Because it was used for so many conditions, it has been called a cure-all. The infusion, made from the entire plant, has been used to treat asthma, whooping cough, gastro-intestinal disorders, premenstrual symptoms, and pain of different origins. It is said to reduce blood pressure and high cholesterol. Dosage: 250 mg capsules up to three times a day. Poultices placed on the skin have been used to treat bruises and heal wounds.

GINSENG – Ginseng, a locally grown herb, is said to top the list of medicinal herbs, because it has so many uses and because it helps both the mind and body. Ginseng, which old-timers called *'sang* is said to be "good for everything that ails you." Specific ailments for which ginseng has been used include asthma, coughs, boils, nervousness, and memory problems. Ginseng is chewed as a great picker-upper. It was also said to be an aphrodisiac. Older roots, if shaped like a human body, were highly treasured. In 1999, dried ginseng was selling in Tennessee for $400 per pound.

HONEY - Never give honey to a child less than two years old. However, its benefits for adults are supposed to be extraordinary.

We often used honey as a sweetener instead of sugar. It was also used as a home remedy for many physical problems.

Honey is believed to kill bacteria and promote healing. In one study, typhoid-producing germs reportedly were put in pure honey, and the germs were dead within 48 hours. Typhus bacteria died within 24 hours, while microorganisms found in bowel feces died within five hours. Pneumonia germs died on the third day. Dysentery-producing germs were dead within ten hours. This information came from bulletin #242 from Colorado Agriculture College in Fort Collins.

Some consider the putty-wax, known as propolis, which bees use as the foundation for honeycomb, to be one of the greatest healers of all time. Propolis and honey have been used to heal frozen toes, which otherwise would be amputated. It has been used to treat burns, tonsillitis, fever, diphtheria, salmonella, herpes, acne, ulcers, influenza, staph, and even cancer. One of my granddaughters used propolis to clear up some acne that plagued her. The results were miraculous.

HYPNOSIS - For many years, I have been interested in the possible medical benefits of hypnosis. My use of hypnosis while on the job almost got me fired, however. A young man came into the Gatlinburg Medical Center early one morning suffering from kidney stones. After giving him what we termed a slug of morphine, he was in such pain that he was running all over the room, and we were not allowed to give him any more medication.

Because I could not bear to watch such horrible suffering, I decided to use hypnosis. Without mentioning the word, I told him if he would get on the bed and do as I said, the medication could help him. With his mother standing beside me, I touched different parts of his body and told him to relax first his feet, then his ankles, legs, hips, and chest. When I touched his face, he just passed out as if asleep. His amazed mother asked what I had done. I did not want him to hear the word h*ypnosis,* so I wrote it on a pad and showed it to her. Seeing her son, with such blessed relief, she replied she did not care what I was using.

About this time, Terrell Tanner, his doctor, arrived. The patient was still quiet, and I realized I needed to tell the doctor what I had done. I told Dr. Tanner that I could not stand to watch the boy suffer any more, so I hypnotized him. He had already seen the patient lying quietly, but you have never seen a doctor explode as he did. He yelled at me that I had better not let word get out that we were using hypnosis at that medical center.

He never mentioned it again, but I later heard that he opened a medical clinic using hypnosis in another state.

LAYING ON OF HANDS - In the *Bible*, people practiced what they called "laying on of hands." Today, a number of hospitals in other parts of the country use Therapeutic Touch, based upon work by Dolores Krieger, which many believe helps to reduce pain, speed the healing of wounds, promote relaxation, and reduce anxiety associated with cancer, heart disease and burns.

I have done what I call "touch therapy." A few people have said my touch therapy has helped them. Once at First Baptist Church in Gatlinburg, Marjorie Chalmers, the head nurse at Pi Beta Phi School for many years, was sitting beside me. She mentioned the terrible arthritic pain in her hands. For some reason, I reached over and held her hands for a few minutes. I said nothing, and I was not doing or thinking anything special as we continued to talk. After Sunday School, she went on to sing in the choir. After church, she found me to tell me that her hands stopped hurting after I held them.

A number of years ago, William Parker held a seminar in Knoxville dealing with Kirlian photography. Although it is a controversial topic, I found it very interesting. Mr. Parker chose me from the audience and photographed my hands using his special Kirlian equipment. First, I stood quietly for perhaps three minutes. Then he snapped a picture of my hands. Then, he asked me to think of the most exciting thing I could imagine, and he snapped a second picture of my hands. Next, he asked me to send "healing thoughts" to someone who was ill.

I have a composite copy of those three pictures. In the first, you can scarcely see the outline of my fingers. In the second picture, one can see a lighted outline. In the third picture, it looks like a light bulb came on.

When attempting touch therapy, I do not actually touch a patient. I start by centering myself and attuning myself with God and the universe. I believe I find pain in someone's body when it feels hot. When I move my hands farther away from the body, it feels like the tip of a cone that is getting smaller. When I move my hands back toward the body, the cone gets larger.

After attempting touch therapy, I have found it is necessary to wash my hands in cold water, because they tend to burn and can remain red and hot for up to two weeks. When that happened to me one time, two people who had witnessed the treatment the night before, saw my red hands the following day.

ONIONS - A universal healing food used to treat colds, fever, earache, diarrhea, warts, lung, liver or intestinal problems. A neighbor mentioned that she heard that Park officials still use raw onion for snakebites. Onion poultices were used like mustard plasters for chest ailments such as bad colds and coughs. To make an onion plaster, onions were baked and mashed into a clean cloth. The plasters were then placed on the bare chest while still hot.

Cut onion is believed to absorb germs in a sick room. For that reason, it is said that one should never use a piece of onion that has been cut and left in the kitchen all day.

PAWPAWS - Our people never cultivated pawpaws, our locally grown bananas, very well. Their aroma in the house was worth their weight in gold. Just a whiff, to me, was as satisfying as a full meal. Used as a cure-all, like our ginseng, we thought they helped with anemia, depression, high blood pressure, constipation, hangovers, heartburn, morning sickness, nerves and ulcers. They have also been used for mosquito bites and for removing warts. Someone even suggested that a banana (pawpaw) a day keeps the doctor away.

PEACH TREES – Tea made from peach leaves is great for upset/sick stomach, vomiting, and diarrhea. Peach trees were used for many medicinal purposes. The leaves are great made into poultices for stone bruises or boils. We bruised peach leaves, bound them on puncture wounds, and expected the wounds to heal quickly. Because we used peach leaves, we were not afraid of tetanus. However, a doctor assured me that we were just lucky.

Our family credits peach tree tea with saving my sister's life. My sister, Gladys [Trentham Russell Yeaton], had a very severe case of measles. She was so sick that water would not stay on her stomach. I overheard my parents whispering that we were going to lose her if something was not done right away. I think they found the suggestion for making peach tree tea in the old Dr. Pierce's medical book. Using peach tree tea, my sister started improving. She was so debilitated that she had to learn to walk all over again. She literally had to tell her feet to move.

As result of that experience, Gladys has made and canned peach tea all her life. We consider it a life-saving elixir. Our daughters even took it to the University of Tennessee when they were roommates as students there. A friend of theirs, who had previously refused peach tree tea, got so "hung-over" while at school that she finally agreed to use it. After her miraculous recovery, she wrote me a letter urging me to put that medication on the market. As a result, my husband Ray and I took a bottle of it to a chemist in Knoxville to learn what we had. He soon came back grinning and told us it was pure cyanide - a deadly poison.

PENNYROYAL – We rubbed pennyroyal on our clothes and skin as an insect repellent when we went to pick berries. However, we did not use pennyroyal tea as some did. In gathering information for this book, I learned that many people used this very common plant to treat indigestion, headaches, kidney and liver ailments, colds, fevers, and coughs. It was also used to promote sweating and to induce menstruation. Perhaps its most controversial use was as an aid for abortions. It is considered dangerous, because of the risk of hemorrhaging. It should obviously never be used during pregnancy, and it is considered dangerous if one is breast-feeding.

PEPPERMINT – has been used for diarrhea, congestion, gas, menstrual cramps, and sore muscles. It can be drunk in tea or applied to the skin. One can also inhale the aroma or a smoke made from the leaves. Peppermint is said to slow or stop the growth of some bacteria.

PRAYER – Prayer has always been considered a great healer in the mountains. It is considered a given that if someone prays for another, the healing hand of God will touch the other person.

We have said that if two people agree to pray for the exact same thing, saying the same words, it multiples the power at least ten times more than if only one person prays.

Years ago, when my husband was the minister at a church in Harriman, I met with a group of women in the church, and we agreed to pray about a situation that we believed was very destructive. Within the week, the man at the center of the problem, dropped dead. That prayer circle came to an abrupt halt.

I have read that following the rules of prayer is important. One must truly believe that it is possible, and one must not be afraid to ask for what is needed. We should picture what we pray for as already happening. For example, seeing a person as being healthy, not sick. What a shame that we have prayed "Lord, bless the sick" while not really expecting any results.

SAGE – Sage has been used to treat diabetes, sore throats, and indigestion. Crushed sage leaves were bound on wounds. Many enjoy drinking it as a tea for a variety of ailments such as colds, flu, headaches, cough, and fever. It has also been used to reduce blood sugar levels and to treat hot flashes.

It is not a favorite of mine, but it has so many uses that it has the reputation for being a cure-all. In fact, a neighbor remarked that no one should ever be sick when sage was growing out back.

SIGNS OF THE MOON – Many in our area believed in using the ancient belief in signs of the moon to help with healing and for planting crops. My husband's parents always discussed when they would plant their crops based upon these signs. According to this belief, a person was more likely to have problems in one area of the body based upon when he or she was born, or they could use various herbal remedies based upon their associations with different body parts.

Each part of the body is associated with a particular moon sign as listed below. When the moon was in a certain constellation, old-timers would say that the signs were in the head, the chest, or other body part. Some signs seem to overlap, but believers seemed to understand.

147

- Aries – head and organs in the head

- Taurus – throat and neck

- Gemini – chest, shoulders, arms and the nervous system

- Cancer – lower chest, breasts, stomach, and digestive system

- Leo - heart, spine, and upper back

- Virgo - digestive system and nervous system

- Libra - kidneys, back, buttocks and skin

- Scorpio – reproductive and excretory systems

- Sagittarius – liver, hips and thighs

- Capricorn – bones, knees, and joints

- Aquarius – circulatory system, ankles, and lower legs

- Pisces - feet, toes, and glands

According to this belief, one should not have elective surgery during the full moon or during the time the moon is in the sign associated with that part of the body. I know a doctor today in this area who says he checks signs of the moon for his patients.

SLIPPERY ELM POWDERS - I cannot say enough good things about slippery elm powders. Slippery elm was used by Native Americans as a poultice for wounds, for digestive problems, and for colds and hay fever. As in most other herbs such as the yellowroot I dug, slippery elm was not brewed. It was put in water overnight, and the water was drunk as a tea. Later we purchased it in powder form. Now it is only available in capsules if you can find it.

As mentioned previously in this book, I have had very good results when I have used it for burns. Used as a poultice, it will draw out boils, carbuncles, or other infections. Mix with Vaseline for longer-lasting poultices or with water for short-term use.

Many report very good results for problems associated with sores in the mouth, such as those under dentures. Dampen a small amount of the powder and put it in dentures to fit over a sore spot. It acts as a cushion. The powder is good for the stomach, so there is no problem with swallowing it.

When I was 60 years old, I asked a pharmacist for slippery elm powder. When he asked me what I intended to do with it, I explained its use for dentures. He told me that slippery elm powder is used for abortions and that he was not allowed to sell it for that purpose. I do not know how they were used. Slippery elm may be found in some health food stores, and pharmacists may be able to special order it.

SASSAFRAS - Tea made of red root sassafras trees is *dee-licious*. Some believe it thins the blood. Chewing a twig calms you down. Sassafras poles make good chicken roosts. It is believed the poles prevent chicken mites.

TURPENTINE – was used for a number of ailments and conditions. When someone had what we called "painter's colic," I understand that turpentine was held to the navel, but I would not recommend it. Turpentine was also used to treat diarrhea and for abortions. When our cows had what was called "hollow-tail" or "hollow-head," my father held turpentine to their navels as a remedy. We were always careful to say that if someone ingested turpentine, it was very important to follow it with castor oil to prevent severe constipation.

VINEGAR – By the time I was growing up, we bought vinegar in the stores in glass bottles. Because we had so many varieties of apples in our orchard, my family probably made their own vinegar before that time. Vinegar has so many uses that it would be nearly impossible to name them all. It is said to have thirty nutrients, a dozen minerals, and over half a dozen vitamins, essential acids, and enzymes. If you look in the index of this book, you will find a very large number of uses for this seemingly miraculous product. I will name a few listed previously in this book: sunburn, sore throat, baldness, flatulence, gout, indigestion, poison ivy, and prevention of senility.

YELLOWROOT - (also called golden seal) has been used for many ailments. Native Americans made a tea from it and used it to treat ulcers in the mouth and stomach as well as for various skin ailments. It has been used for sore throat, indigestion, diarrhea, Crohn's disease, and as a tonic. The FDA does not approve its use, but I have seen enough success with it to believe that it can be genuinely helpful.

The yellowroot plant grows near water. I often dug roots for my mother, who cleaned them and put them in water. Letting the water and root set overnight, she sometimes drank the resulting liquid for indigestion or stomach problems. Today, I buy the capsules, open them, and put the contents in water. It is a very refreshing drink for upset stomach.

CONCLUSION

Over the last 85 years, I have used many remedies mentioned in this book with good results. I have seen some that have made no difference at all, and there are some I would never even consider. I collected ideas from neighbors and friends, who may or may not have used some of the remedies they described. Those who shared their memories seemed to enjoy the opportunity. I thank them again for their wonderful contributions.

I have enjoyed collecting and compiling all these remedies and remembering the stories that went along with many of them. I feel as if I have put together a life's work here. It reminds me of a time when life was much simpler than today. I hope all of this has been equally enjoyable for you. Just as importantly, I hope you have learned more about the people of the Smoky Mountains.

INDEX

Abortion 96
Abscesses 138
Acne 29, 138, 140
Age spots...............................30
Aging......................................30
Albumen poisoning.................57
Alcohol
    baldness 31
    drinking problems.............42
    poisoning 73
Alfalfa
    arthritis.............................24
    general uses 136
    tonic...................................21
    urinary infections.............58
Allergies 101
Allspice
    diarrhea.............................46
    flatulence 47
Almonds
    cancer.................................55
Aloe
    baldness 32
    burns 117
    frostbite............................120
    shingles.............................124
Alum
    blood poisoning..................61
Aluminum
    Alzheimer's.......................84
    deodorants..........................36
Alzheimer's disease................84
Ammonia
    insect bites 88
Anemia............................60, 144
Anger......................................76
Anise
    epilepsy.............................77
Antacids
    alcohol consumption.........42
Ants 86

Aphrodisiac 139
Appendicitis 43, 138
Apples
    constipation 44
    pink eye 134
    urinary infections...............58
Arsenic poisoning....................73
Arthritis 23, 136, 137
Asafetida 136
Aspirin
    bee sting.............................89
    shingles.............................124
    sunburn 125
Asthma 11, 102, 139
Athlete's foot 114
Baby
    food...................................18
    nursing...............................16
Baby powder
    burns 116
Bacon fat
    boils and carbuncles 114
Baking soda.............................49
    acne....................................29
    alcohol consumption............42
    athlete's foot 114
    baldness 31
    bathing baby 16
    burns 117
    deodorant 36
    foot odor 37
    indigestion 49
    insect bites 89
    shingles.............................124
    skin rash............................123
    sore throat.........................111
    stop smoking.......................51
    sunburn 124
    tooth paste..........................34
Baldness 31
Bandages 71

Bathing 32
Bayberry
   chapped hands 118
   general uses 136
   hemorrhoids 48
   mouthwash 33
   varicose veins 38
Bayberry bark
   circulation 61
Bearberry 56
Bedbugs 87
Bed-wetting 16
Bee pollen
   impotence 98
Bees
   arthritis 25
Beet juice
   nose drops 106
Belladonna
   whooping cough 67
Benson, Ray 95
Bible verse
   bleeding 59
Birth 15
Birth control 96
Birthing stool 14
Black cohosh 97
   coughs 108
   cramps 97
   female problems 97
   whooping cough 68
Black Drought
   constipation 43
Black walnut
   bruises 115
   ringworm 91
   scabies 122
Blackberry
   diarrhea 46
   healing sores 119
Blood
   clots 61, 138
   poisoning 61
   pressure 139, 144

purifier 137
stopper 9
sugar 56, 147
sugar 136
thinner 150
Bloodroot
   eczema 120
   poison oak 91
   scabies 122
   skin problems 113
Blowing out the fire 116
Blueberries
   night blindness 133
Boils .. 11, 114, 138, 139, 144, 149
Bold hives 9
Bones, broken 70
Boneset
   colds and flu 105
   constipation 44
   spring tonic 21
   typhoid fever 67
Boyer, Ed. 125
Brandy
   lung cancer 55
   sinus problems 110
   tuberculosis 112
Bras
   cancer 55
Bread
   fishbone 46
Bronchitis 103, 138
Brown sugar
   cataracts 132
Bruises 115
Buckeyes 7
   rheumatism 24
Burdock
   blood purifier 61
   eczema 120
   general uses 137
   measles 65
   psoriasis 123
Burn doctor 10, 116
Burns 116

Buttermilk
  age spots 30
  asthma................................ 103
  diarrhea.............................. 45
Cabbage
  alcohol consumption............. 42
  pin worms 90
  ulcers 51
Camphor
  rheumatism 24
  Snake oil.............................. 5
Cancer 53, 54
  dogwood............................. 54
  honey 140
  lungs 55
  Stomach 55
  touch therapy 142
Canker sores 137
Caraway
  epilepsy.............................. 77
Carbuncles..................... 114, 149
Carrot
  cancer................................. 55
Carter's Little Liver Pills........... 58
Castor oil 4, 36
  age spots 30
  appendicitis........................ 43
  baldness 31
  childbirth 15
  children.............................. 13
  corns and calluses............... 118
  digestive concerns 42
  eye lashes........................... 37
  eyes.................................... 36
  granulated eyelids............... 132
  indigestion 49
  pink eye 134
Cataracts............................... 131
Catnip
  bronchitis 103
  chicken pox.......................... 64
  colic 18
  diarrhea.............................. 46
  hives 19

hot flashes.......................... 97
  indigestion 49
Cayce, Edgar 112
  arthritis.............................. 26
  TB...................................... 112
Celery
  high blood pressure 62
Cellulite................................ 33
Certo
  arthritis.............................. 25
Chalmers
  Marjorie................. 3, 63, 142
Chamomile 137
  general uses 137
  hair color........................... 30
  hot flashes.......................... 97
  indigestion 50
  insomnia 82
  mouth odor 33
  pink eye 134
Chapped hands 118
Charcoal
  flatulence 47
  food poisoning..................... 48
  indigestion 47
Cherries
  gout.................................... 27
Chest congestion 103
Chestnut leaves
  frostbite.............................. 120
Chicken pox 64, 138
Chickens............................. 128
Chiggers 87
Chihuahua - dog
  asthma............................... 103
Chives
  high blood pressure 62
Cholera................................ 138
Cholesterol 136, 139
Cinnamon 56
  arthritis.............................. 25
  bed-wetting......................... 17
  diabetes.............................. 56
  diarrhea.............................. 45

157

urinary infection 58
Circulation 137
Citrus fruits
    bruises 116
Clay
    cast 70
    facial 39
Cloves
    blood clotting 61
    diabetes 56
    insect bites 89
    toothache 34
    wounds 74
Coal tar soap
    shampoo 113
    skin problems 113
Cobwebs
    bleeding 60
    wounds 74
Coca-Cola
    sore throat 111
    vomiting 51
Cod liver oil
    blood thinner 17
    children 17
Coffee
    hair color 30
Colds and flu 17, 104, 136, 138,
    143, 147
Colgate Toothpaste
    shingles 124
Colic 18
Congestion 146
Conjunctivitis 11
Constipation 43, 136, 144
Corn
    warts 126
Corn oil
    asthma 103
    hairballs 128
Cornmeal
    dry shampoo 38
Corns and calluses 118
Cornsilk

bed-wetting 17
Cornstarch
    dry shampoo 38
    shingles 124
Coughs 107, 139, 147
Cows 128
Cradle cap 18, 139
Cranberry
    urinary infection 58
Crohn's Disease 44
Cucumber
    black eyes 131
    burns 117
    facial 39
    hot flashes 98
    puffy eyes 36
Cutex nail polish remover
    shingles 124
Cylinder oil
    baldness 31
    mange 129
Dandelion
    corns and calluses 118
Dental Care 33
Deodorants 35
Depression 11, 144
Diabetes 55, 56
Diapers 16
Diarrhea .. 10, 11, 45, 46, 136, 143,
    144, 146, 151
Dill
    hot flashes 97
Diphtheria 65, 140
Diuretic 136
Doan's Backache Kidney Pills .. 26
Dog days 119
Dog hobble
    itch 122
Dogs 129
Dogwood
    cancer 54
Drano
    predicting baby's sex 20
Dropsy 61

158

Duct tape
 warts 126
Dunn, Andrew 125
Dysentery 9
Earache 108, 143
Echinacea
 acne 30
 appendicitis 43
 boils 115
 chicken pox 64
 colds and flu 104
 eczema 120
 general uses 137
 headache 81
 mastitis 19
 measles 65
 poison ivy 91
 snakebite 92
 tonsillitis 112
 typhoid fever 67
 ulcers 52
Eczema 119, 137
Eggwhite
 facial 39
 spider bite 93
Elderberry
 colds and flu 105
Elmer's Glue-all
 warts 126
Epilepsy 77
Epsom salts 4
 bee sting 88
 blood clots 138
 general uses 138
 ingrown toenails 121
 insect bites 88
 shingles 124
Ether 5
Ethridge, David 106
Evening primrose
 asthma 103
 blood pressure 62, 139
 cradle cap 18
 general uses 139

indigestion 50
menstrual problems 98
whooping cough 68
Eyes 36
 black 131
 color 36
 lashes 37
Fainting 11, 78
Fatigue 56
Feeble-minded 79
Feet
 burning 119
 cold 118
Felons 120
Female problems 97
Fennel tea
 colic 18
Fever 138, 147
Fever blisters, cold sores 119
Feverfew
 headache 80
Fishbone 46
Flannigan, William 127
Flatulence 46, 146
Flaxseeds 54
 boils and carbuncles 114
 cows 129
 diabetes 56
 eyes 132
 psoriasis 123
 tonsilitis 111
 warts 126
Flu 147
Food Poisoning 47
Foot odor 37
Freckles 11, 37
Frostbite 120
Fumigation 64
Gallstones 10
Garlic
 cold germs 107
 colds and flu 104
 high blood pressure 62
 wounds 74

159

Geranium
    shingles 124
Gin
    rheumatism 24
Ginger
    arthritis............................... 25
    burns 117
    coughs................................ 107
    indigestion 47
Ginseng
    anemia 60
    asthma................................ 103
    general uses 139
    impotence 98
    senility 84
    stress 84
Glycerin................................. 124
Goiter
    iodine 57
Golden Medical Discovery 7
    tuberculosis........................ 112
    whooping cough 67
Golden seal .... *See* Yellowroot
Grape vine
    baldness 31
Grapes
    energy 57
Grouchiness............................. 80
Gunpowder
    blood poisoning 61
Hair care 37
Hairballs, cats......................... 128
Hangovers 144, 145
Headaches 80, 138, 147
Healers...................................... 4
Heart
    cod liver oil......................... 17
Heartburn 144
Hemorrhoids............... 11, 48, 137
Henderson, Dr. Joe.................... 74
Hepatitis 65
Hiccoughs............................... 48
Hickory
    hair color............................ 30

Hippoed 81
Hives 19, 121
Hoarseness............................. 109
Hoffman, Dr. 3
Hollow horn 128, 150
Honey 43, 56, 140
    age spots 31
    allergies 102
    arthritis............................... 24
    baldness 32
    bed-wetting......................... 16
    burns 117
    colds and flu 107
    diabetes............................... 56
    energy 57
    general uses 139
    heart problems 61
    hoarseness......................... 109
    hot flashes.......................... 97
    ingrown toenails 121
    insomnia 82
    night blindness.................... 133
    sore throat.......................... 111
Honeycomb 140
    respiratory ailments 110
Horehound weed
    poison ivy 91
Hornet's nest
    frostbite.............................. 120
Horseradish
    bronchitis 103
    hoarseness......................... 109
Hot flashes.............................. 97
Hydrogen peroxide
    age spots 30
    gum problems 34
    skunk odor 130
Hypnosis................................ 140
Ichthammol
    skin problems 115
Impotence................................ 98
Indigestion.......... 49, 137, 149, 151
Insect bites.............................. 88
Insomnia........................... 82, 137

In-toeing 27
Iodine
   baldness 31
   colds and flu 106
   goiter.................................... 57
   thyroid function 57
   tonsilitis 112
Iridology................................. 20
Itching 121, 137
Ivy, ground
   colic 18
Jimson weed
   eye color 36
Kerosene
   bedbugs................................ 87
   body lice 90
   chickens 128
   chiggers 87
   cuts 71
   diptheria.............................. 65
   hemorrhoids.......................... 48
   whooping cough 68
Kerr, Howard 88, 91
Kidney.................................... 57
Krieger, Dolorous.................... 142
Lameness
   animals............................... 130
   people 27
Lard
   chiggers 88
   corns and calluses.............. 118
Laxative...................... 136, 138
Laying on of hands.................. 142
Leeks
   burns 117
Legs
   cramps 27
Lemons
   acne.................................... 30
   age spots 30
   dandruff.............................. 33
   facial 39
   felons 120
   fish bone 46

LeQuire, Gene........................... 91
Lice
   body..................................... 90
Licorice
   indigestion 50
lightning 71
Limejuice
   indigestion 47
Linseeds.................See Flaxseeds
Liver....................................... 58
Lye poisoning........................... 73
Mad dogs (hydrophobia).........127
Magnets
   muscle pain........................... 27
Maples
   Allie Newman................... 108
   Bruce 108
Mare's carry 10
Masturbation 99
Materia medica 6
McMahan, Dr. 2
Measles........................65, 138
Meat tenderizer
   bee sting............................... 89
Melaleuca oil
   bee sting............................... 89
Memory 139
Menstrual cramps 146
Mental
   mental illness 83
   mentally unsound................. 12
Merthiolate
   sinus problems 110
Milk
   puffy eyes 36
   ulcers 52
Milk thistle
   hepatitis 65
Milk weed................................ 19
Molasses, and sulfur
   spring tonic 21
Moonshine
   baldness 31
Morning sickness 144

Mosquito bites 144
Mullein
    tuberculosis........................... 112
Muscles
    relaxing............................... 138
    sore 146
Mustard
    back pain............................... 27
    tuberculosis........................... 112
Myers
    Amanda Ray 8
    Bess 80
    Bonnie Lynn Trentham......... 53
    Bruce and Ida..................... 147
    Donald Trent.............. 101, 114
    Donna Chesney Barringer .. 114
    Glenn Leland 117
    Ida Jane Headrick 29, 66, 86,
      102, 104
    Ray T 66, 75, 78, 86, 145
    William Bruce 86
Nail polish
    chiggers 88
Nervous stomach..................... 137
Nervousness 139
Newburn, Dr............................. 46
Night blindness........................ 133
Nitro-muriatic
    freckles 37
Nosebleeds 62
Nux Vomica 15
Oatmeal
    facial 39
    shingles.............................. 124
    skin rash............................. 123
Obesity 50
Ogle
    Charles............................... 127
    Dr. John 3
    Ephraim 131
    Mary Jane 30
Olive oil
    cradle cap............................. 18
Onion

bronchitis 103
bruises................................... 115
colds and flu 104
coughs................................... 108
eyes....................................... 132
general uses 143
hair color.............................. 30
ingrown toenails 121
insect bites 89
pneumonia 109
sickroom 64
snakebite............................... 92
splinters 73
warts 126
Orange peel
    age spots 30
Outhouses................................. 65
Painter's colic......................... 150
Paregoric
    colic 18
Parker, William 142
Parsley
    epilepsy................................ 77
    mouth odor 33
    prevent insect bites 89
    sties..................................... 134
Pawpaws
    bee sting............................... 89
    bruises................................. 115
    constipation 44
    hair color.............................. 30
    hangover............................... 43
    morning sickness 98
    stress 84
    ulcers 52
    warts 126
Peach
    baldness 31
    black eyes 131
    constipation 44
    general uses 144
    healing sores 119
    indigestion 50
    tetanus........................... 73, 144

Pemberton, Luella 54
Pendulum
    baby's sex 20
Pennyroyal
    abortions 146
    chiggers 87
    colds 146
    colds and flu 106
    coughs................................ 146
    dangers 146
    fevers 146
    general uses 145
    headaches..................... 81, 146
    indigestion 49, 146
    kidney problems 58
Peony
    Epilepsy 77
Pepper........................... 5, 45
    ants 86
    arthritis.............................. 24
    baldness 31
    blood thinner...................... 61
    bronchitis 103
    cold feet........................... 118
    colds and flu 104, 107
    diarrhea.............................. 45
    headache 80
    hoarseness......................... 109
    hollow horn 129
    pneumonia 110
    shingles............................. 124
    sore throat......................... 111
    toothache 34
Peppermint
    colds and flu 107
    Crohn's disease 45
    diarrhea.............................. 46
    general uses 146
    indigestion 47
    menstrual problems 98
    mouth odor 33
Persimmon
    ringworm 92
Phillips Milk of Magnesia

shingles............................... 124
Pi Beta Phi School.................... 63
Pickle, Robert.......................... 32
Pickles
    food poisoning..................... 47
Pierce, Dr. Ray Vaughn .6, 65, 66,
    67, 112, 122, 145
Pin worms............................... 90
Pine
    colds and flu 107
    warts 125
Pinkeye-conjunctivitis............. 134
Pleasant Pellets
    scabies 122
Pneumonia...................... 109, 140
Podophyllum
    warts 126
Poison ivy.............................. 138
Poisons 72
Poke
    Mastitis 19
    scabies 122
Pokeroot
    poison ivy 91
Pollen
    energy 57
Potato
    arthritis.............................. 24
    asthma.............................. 103
    black eyes 131
    boils and carbuncles 115
    diabetes............................ 56
    eczema............................ 119
    hemorrhoids....................... 48
    pink eye 134
    warts 126
Prayer 146
Pregnancy............................... 95
    overdue 10
Premature labor 138
Premenstrual symptoms 98, 139
Preparation H
    acne................................. 30
    puffy eyes 36

varicose veins 38
Propolis 55, 140
   acne.................................... 29
   burns 117
   diphtheria............................ 65
   frostbite................................ 120
   ingrown toenails 121
   mastitis................................ 19
   open wounds....................... 74
   tonsillitis 112
Psoriasis........................... 123, 137
Pumpkin
   impotence 98
   urinary infection 57
Queen of the Meadow
   kidney 58
Quinsy (tonsilitis)................... 111
Rabies.................................... 137
Ragweed
   insect bites 89
Raisin
   rheumatism 24
   toothache 34
Rash....................................... 123
Reagan, Richard 72
Red cabbage
   coughs................................ 107
Red clover 55
   coughs................................ 107
Rheumatism.............. 23, 136, 137
Rhubarb
   pin worms 90
Ringworm................................ 92
Robertson, Jessica 96
Rock candy
   coughs................................ 108
   hoarseness........................... 109
Rosemary
   hair color............................. 30
Sage
   diabetes............................... 56
   general uses 147
   hair color............................. 30
   hot flashes............................ 97

indigestion 49
sore throat........................... 111
wounds 74
Salmonella............................. 140
Salt water
   colds and flu 106
Sassafras................................ 150
   blood thinner....................... 61
Sauerkraut juice
   hangover 43
Scabies (The itch)................... 122
Scarlet fever 138
Senility 84
Sen-Sen
   mouth odor 32
Sex
   drive................................... 10
   unborn baby........................ 19
Shilling, Dr. Ralph .. 7, 47, 51, 119
Shingles.................................. 123
Shortening, vegetable
   skin moisturizer 118
Signs of the moon.................... 147
Sinus headaches 111
Skin diseases 113
Skunk odor 130
Slippery elm
   abortion................................ 97
   baby food............................ 19
   boils and carbuncles 115
   burns 117
   dentures 35
   general uses 149
   indigestion 50
   wounds 74
Slugs
   itching................................ 121
Smelling salts
   fainting................................ 78
Snake oil................................... 5
Snakebites 92, 137, 138, 143
Soap....................................... 32
   acid burns 117
   leg cramps........................... 28

Sore throat 147
Sores....................................... 137
Sourwood tree
   asthma................................ 102
Spicewood
   spring tonic 21
Spider bites.............................. 93
Splinters................................... 73
Sprains..................................... 138
Spring tonic 21
Stanback Headache Powders..... 80
Staphylococcus........................ 140
Sties... 134
Stogner, Kate Trentham 3, 63
Stone bruises 144
Stress 84
Sugar
   hiccups.................................. 49
   open wounds......................... 74
Sulfur
   bedbugs................................ 87
   blood poisoning.................... 61
   scabies 122
   spring tonic 21
Sun blindness 134
Sunburn 124
Sunflower
   impotence 98
   sun blindness 134
Surgery.................................... 5
Sweet oil (olive oil)
   corns and calluses............... 118
   earache................................ 108
   frostbite............................... 120
Syphilis.............................. 9, 138
Tanner, Dr. Terrell 7, 141
Tea bags
   puffy eyes 36
Teething ring............................ 16
Tetanus 73
Tetter 113
Throat obstruction 21
Thrush 22
Ticks.. 94

Tobacco 51
   insect bites 88
   snakebite.............................. 93
   snuff.................................... 15
Toenails, ingrown.................... 121
Toilet tissue 66
Tomato juice
   pink eye 134
   poison ivy 91
   skunk odor 130
Tomatoes
   burning feet......................... 119
Tonic 136
Tonsillitis................ 111, 138, 140
Toothache................................ 137
Touch therapy......................... 142
Trentham
   Ben 79
   Harmon................................ 63
   Mary Jane Ogle Carr ... 3, 5, 14,
     69, 85, 95, 122, 123, 127
   Noah H. 2, 6, 44, 45, 58, 69, 79,
     128
   Ollie.................................... 123
   Robert Lee 43
   Sam................................. 69, 85
   Sophia.................................. 112
   William Thomas 43
   Wilson 123
Tuberculosis 11, 112
Turpentine 45
   abortion................................ 96
   cod liver oil.......................... 17
   colds and flu 106
   cuts 71
   diarrhea................................ 45
   digestive concerns 42
   frostbite............................... 121
   general uses 150
   hollow horn 128
   lameness 27, 130
   painter's colic 150
   pneumonia 110
   snakebite.............................. 92

Turpentine 150
Tyler, Mrs. Guilford (Thelma) .. 13
Typhoid 66, 140
Ulcers 51, 138, 144
Ultrasound 19
Urinary tract infection 136
Urine
   earache 109
Vanilla
   tongue 117
Vapors 78, 97
Varicose veins 38
Vaseline
   baldness 31
Vinegar 61
   age spots 31
   alcohol consumption 42
   ammonia poisoning 72
   arthritis 24
   baldness 32
   burns and sunburn 117
   cataracts 132
   corns and calluses 118
   dandruff 33
   deodorant 35
   energy 57
   facial 39
   flatulence 47
   food poisoning 47
   general uses 150
   gout 27
   gum problems 34
   hair rinse 33
   headache 80
   hoarseness 109
   hot flashes 97
   insect bites 89
   insomnia 82
   lameness 27
   lameness 130
   leg cramps 27
   poison ivy 91
   pregnant cows 129
   puffy eyes 36

   ringworm 92
   scabies 122
   senility 84
   shampoo 38
   shingles 124
   sickroom 64
   skin rash 123
   sore throat 111
   sprains 28
   sunburn 124
   weight loss 51
   wounds 74
   yeast infection 99
Violet
   grouchiness 80
   spring tonic 21
Vitamin E
   age spots 30
Vomiting 51
Wallace, Annie 41
Walnut
   hair color 30
   shingles 123
Warts 143, 144
   charming 125
Water
   purifying 67
Watkins liniment
   hollow horn 129
Watson, Lillie Trentham ... 57, 102
WD-40
   arthritis 26
   corns and calluses 119
   mange 129
   mosquito bites 89
Whiskey
   coughs 108
   food poisoning 48
   itching 121
   pneumonia 110
White-eyed 78
Whooping cough 67, 139
Wild cherry tree
   coughs 108

Wintergreen
    mouth odor 33
Witch hazel
    cold sores 119
    dandruff 33
    facial 39
    frostbite 120
    menstrual problems 98
    shingles 124
    varicose veins 38
Wood pulp
    cancer 55
Wounds 130, 147

Wrinkles 38
Yeast infection 99
Yeaton, Gladys Trentham Russell
    .... 2, 69, 83, 145
Yellowroot 44, 151
    cold sores 119
    Crohn's disease 151
    general uses 151
    indigestion 49
Yogurt
    burns 117
Zinc
    colds and flu 104

www.ingramcontent.com/pod-product-compliance
Lightning Source LLC
LaVergne TN
LVHW011352080426
835511LV00005B/250